An Intimate Journey Overcoming Agoraphobia

An Intimate Journey
Overcoming Agoraphobia

Sharon McCarthy

One Spirit Press
Portland, Oregon

ISBN: 978-1-893075-93-1

Library of Congress Control Number: 2011934420

Cover Design and Original Art Ethan Firpo
Book Design Spirit Press, LLC

One Spirit Press
www.onespiritpress.com
onespiritpress@gmail.com

Publishers Note

The Original title of the book was *Flight of a Dove and A Broken Wing*. We found the title wonderful. But, we were unsure if those needing this work would find it with the first title, so the title was changed. However, we felt the Flight of a Dove was an appropriate description of Ms. McCarthy's Journey. We sincerely hope this special and intimate work will help you or a loved one in their journey.

FLIGHT OF A DOVE
and
A broken wing
The Dove being symbolic of us all
As we journey through this lifetime

The broken wing is symbolic of our
Struggles through our lessons

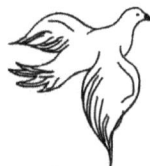

Table of Contents

Dedication

To my husband Dennis

When you were supportive, it was wonderful!
And when you couldn't be, I learned about me

And so, in being who you are, it inspired
although, sometimes painfully, the growth
that I have seen in me.

I am forever grateful with love
You are still the best!

and

To my children Justin, Todd and Evan

I am very proud of each one of you
and I love you with all my heart!

You are the light of my life!

and

To my Mother who raised seven children
and survived the challenges

and

In memory of my Father and his final years of sobriety.

God Bless!

A Word of Thanks

I would like to thank the many people with whom I chose to share or critique my manuscript, whose invaluable comments culminated in my preparing a book of international scope. There is a special place in my heart for my friends Melissa and Deborah, for their technical support at a moment's notice, and their enthusiasm and encouragement when it was most critical. I owe a special word of gratitude to James A. Doss for his many hours of computer mentoring and essentially holding my hand as I approached the finish line. Also, thanks to James for his domestic and global marketing expertise, his knowledge of business and contracts. A special thank you to Suzanne Deakins and One Spirit Press. I am so grateful! We share a dream of overseeing a global foundation to provide water and other essentials for those in dire need, and to restore planet Earth during this, our small window of opportunity. I hope this book will provide a cornerstone for the world to partake in such a glorious and miraculous realization. In final thanks I submit to the Holy Spirit, without Whose beautiful inspiration this book would not have been written. I pray He take it along now to where He wants it to go.

Foreword

In March of 1983 I was admitted to Spofford Hall in New Hampshire, a treatment center for family members of alcoholics. At the time there was not a lot published or written about agoraphobia. This was the beginning of my long and arduous journey through recovery from this dilemma.

It was another ten years before I completely recovered and was free of the bondage to fear. I researched, and actively took part in my own healing through many different avenues of treatment, counseling, and spiritual studies. I hope, in sharing what worked for me, that others will benefit and be able to take their lives back. It is a debilitating, confusing, and sometimes paralyzing condition.

Once understood and dealt with through the correct treatment, it is possible to overcome the anxiety and panic, free of drugs, and to be emotionally, physically, and spiritually where you were meant to be.

"Pain has a way of clipping our wings and keeping us from being able to fly, and if it is left unresolved for a very long time, we almost forget that we were meant to fly in the first place."

~Anonymous

Introduction

An Intimate Journey Overcoming Agoraphobia

"For we were not given the spirit of fear-but of love, and of power, and of a sound mind"

~2 Timothy: 1:7

Why is it that some people can go through life unscathed from their circumstances, without so much as a backward glance? And then there are others... We have a journey of endurance and overcoming that consumes our very existence. If we are open to it, we learn life's lessons and simple truths. We surrender and stop complicating things. We begin to learn that it is not what we experience or attain in life that defines our success, but in how we overcome our challenges and adversity. Our bodies follow our mind. The way we view our circumstances determines our emotional, physical, and spiritual wellbeing. We forgive our past and then the healing comes.

Agoraphobia comes from the Greek word *agora* meaning "fear of the marketplace." However, in recent years, it has become much more prevalent in the clinical sense. Millions of people are experiencing panic and anxiety. As a society, we have become socially disconnected from one another. Programs of social networking and internet chatting don't really bring us closer and have a built-in safety barrier where our true nature never needs to be revealed. In a very real sense they isolate us.

We have become prisoners in our own homes. Physical symptoms are very real, overwhelming and, at times, paralyzing. It is a combination of complex symptoms that renders a victim hostage to their emotions, imagined or (real) physical occurrences, which chain you to a cycle of feeding fear-into-fear.

The brain is very complex and intricately connected to our emotions. When a person feels safe, panic subsides. It became evident to me that we can control these physical symptoms by the way we think.

When we are experiencing panic and anxiety, there is a very real physiological response. There is a rush of adrenaline, which can keep a person spinning on a physical and emotional rollercoaster. It feels as if one is having a heart attack or dying. There is an array of physical and emotional symptoms it can be terrifying. We sometimes feel as if we are losing our minds!

Agoraphobia is an all-consuming irrational fear. It is a fear of leaving one's home. It is consistent with panic disorders, phobias of physical illness or phobias of driving- flying- shopping- supermarkets- elevators. It is any irrational fear that borders on obsession.

There is a very real physical occurrence of neuro-chemistry. It is almost like a pinball machine going into tilt. The brain misfires and sends messages that cause malfunction. This comes about as result of the way we view our world or our circumstances.

The feelings of panic tend to self-perpetuate and spiral according to our way of looking at things. One becomes conditioned to the fear that is so vividly imagined. Our brains, over time, become conditioned to the fight-or-flight response.

Panic attacks usually begin without warning, they come out of the blue. They last from a few minutes to several hours and will subside once a person feels safe. Experiencing a panic attack can be one of the most frightening experiences of a person's life. One begins to retreat to limit the physical symptoms and experience of panic. To feel safe, to cocoon themselves in a protective and less threatening environment.

Agoraphobia is a conditioned reaction to the fight-or-flight response (defend or run). When you first experience panic outside in the world your heart is racing, you are dizzy, you become weak, it is terrifying, Consequently you will begin to avoid: wherever you were at the time, whatever you were doing, whoever you were with, erroneously connecting this to your feelings of dread. Thus begins the cycle of feeding fear-into-fear. The merry go round of feelings, thoughts, and emotions that bring on the panic attacks never end until one begins to break this cycle by reeducating their thinking about their life and their circumstances. It is a vicious cycle.

It is a learned response. Ultimately, you become a prisoner to a biochemistry gone into overdrive. Your life becomes a virtual nightmare. Panic and anxiety attacks are a result of this adrenaline rush that is pumped into the bloodstream, causing blood pressure to rise, elevated pulse and shortness of breath. Hyperventilation occurs because you feel as if you cannot breathe, bringing about a total loss of self control. This rush of adrenaline in turn affects the neurons in the brain. They misfire and send conflicting messages that result in the feelings of panic and anxiety.

Successful treatment includes desensitization by facing the fear and by gradual exposure, changing diet, eliminating caffeine, msg, aspartame, several medications, and most important what I call pro-active therapy: cognitive and behavioral therapy with a trusted support person, learning to change your thinking.

My struggle with agoraphobia blessed me with a whole new way of looking at life. I am grateful! This is the story of my journey...

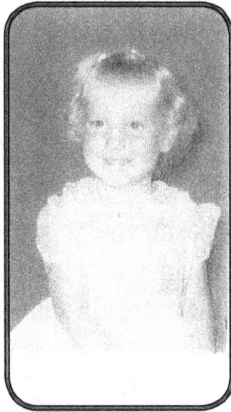

I Believe In The Sun Even When It Is Not Shining

I Believe In Love Even When Not Feeling It

I Believe In God Even When he Is Silent

Anonymous

The Promise Of The Dove In Flight

God is aware of our every breath…He is as close as the
air we breath
The universe whispered to our soul, the moment we were born…
and we heard its thoughts
And we knew the truth and the purpose…as these words were
imparted to us….
I give you life to do as you choose…go forward my child….and
may you come back to me as free as a "Dove in Flight" and feel as
pure as the white glistening snow
I will love you all through your journey, even though you may fall,
and your wings will be bruised, I have given you the capacity to fly
higher each time
And your wings will become stronger each time until you soar!
I just ask that you remember me….and know that you are
loved……..
For it is I that gave you life and the opportunity to feel the wind,
and hear your heart beat, and see the sky in which you fly!

Sharon Reed McCarthy

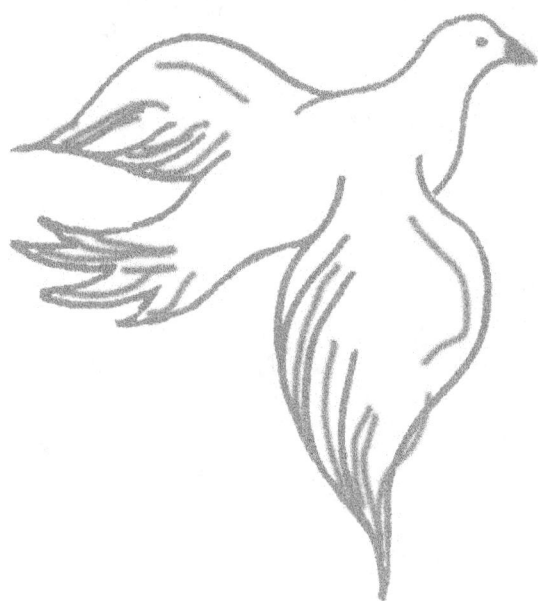

"One is never deceived. One deceives one's self."

~Johanne Wolfgang Van Goethe

The Beginning

I suppose I should bring you back to the beginning. It is 1951 and I was born in Springfield, Massachusetts, into a large Catholic family. My father was English and Irish, and my mother was German and Scotch, although my mother's grandparents were Jewish, but we did not know that then. I grew up the middle of seven children: four girls and three boys. We grew up comfortable. My parents were hard working. We went to parochial schools and had big family holidays: Easter, Thanksgiving, and lots of gifts at Christmas.

When I look back at family photos, we were always well dressed. I remember firm discipline. Today the discipline would be considered too firm. My father was also an alcoholic, but we did not know this at the time. I do not think the term alcoholic was even used back then, unless one was homeless and living on the street. It was such a part of our culture, people drank and smoked everywhere, even in the afternoon at the office, imagine.

When my father was sober, he was very loving and kind. He worked very hard trying to provide for a family of seven children. My mother worked hard and took care of business in the home with firmness and love as well. Together my parents owned and managed a restaurant and catering business. This proved to be a challenge for my parents, and it brought a lot of financial difficulty and heartache to them, especially to my father in later years. I grew up and went through the usual rebellion in my teen years in the sixties. I did experiment with alcohol and drugs, though not as much as others that I knew at the time.

I went on to marry two men that were alcoholics, and had three boys: two from my first marriage and one from my second. I was a perfectionist with a lot of issues from my dysfunctional way of looking at the world. Little did I realize that much of my growth would come through my experiences with my second husband, whom I adored. I, also, had a very ambivalent relationship with him because of his drinking.

My first parochial school memory is on the first day of kindergarten. I am walking down what appears to me to be a very wide, imposing hallway. The marble steps are slippery, and the nuns and priests seem strict and stern. This makes me uncomfortable, but my mother, holding my hand, assures me that everything will be fine. We enter a large classroom bustling with other children my age. My mother comforts me and with a loving smile, kisses me good bye. The nun who is my teacher points to a desk and orders me to sit down. She is not smiling. She is not friendly or welcoming. She is frightening to me.

I scan the room and notice that in the back of the class is a miniature size nun sitting very still. After questioning my senses for a few moments, I determine that she is indeed a real person. What is she doing sitting back there? And why does she look so young? I continue to peek under my arm.

This is very curious to me. Later, I become aware of the fact that the miniature nun, with the miniature face, was also a student, posing as a nun. I suppose this was the teacher's way of discovering which of her students were observant and precocious. Wasn't that innovative?! Things are not always what they appear to be.

As a child, I did not question these innocent and fun occurrences. However, as I grew older, there were a lot of incidents regarding religion, family, and relationships, with life in general, that were much more serious and life altering. Events, experiences, and teachings that were also not what they appeared to be. I still do not question the validity of truth in this life of mine, until I had no choice.

The nuns and priests taught with a no nonsense approach. We were told that God was a punishing God, but that He loved us. Suffering was part of this life, because this is how we learned our lessons. Our parents were made in God's image. So, of course, to a child this is gospel. This is how you begin to see the world and you develop an unshakable trust in your parents, role models, and teachings-- After all, they are made in God's image. How can anything they say or do be anything but absolute *fact?* --And so it goes.

My mother kept a clean and comfortable home. I remember her sewing outfits for us on special occasions. She was also a great cook! My father had his building projects and would create beautiful wood crafts and flower gardens. He lined our yard with lovely brick walks that surrounded our home. He was a musician and played the saxophone in a band on the weekends to supplement the family income. When we were younger, my dad worked as an advertising director for J.C. Penny. Later, they would buy a family restaurant.

In the summers, we would splash carelessly with unrestrained laughter and abandon in our back yard pool.

We would ride our bikes late into the evening. The entire neighborhood would play hide and seek, much to the consternation of the adults, as we jumped their fences and ran across their nicely landscaped lawns. We did not listen as they pleaded and lectured about the disrespect of it all. No matter, we were having a grand old time!

We took long summer vacations to Alexandria, Virginia to visit my grandparents on my Dad's side. We traveled to Maine and frolicked in the ocean, soaking up the sun as the salt water splashed on our face. We watched my mother and father surf the waves in their black inner tube as we built sand castles. Life seemed good!

At Our Lady of the Sacred Heart parochial school, the nuns often slapped and disciplined the students for the slightest infraction, telling us how unruly we were. I developed a sense of wanting to be perfect, so as not to be the focus of their disapproval and wrath. At home, among my six brothers and sisters, I developed the same approach. I wanted to please the people that were important to me. I did not want to disappoint my parents, or the nuns, or the God in heaven, who I could not see. But, he can see me, and he is looking down upon us at all times. Holy terror! It was not until my teen years that I broke out of this illusion and began to rebel.

When I was twelve years old, my father's drinking increased and the progression of the disease becomes evident in his unreasonable discipline and erratic behavior. Impressions and memories of dysfunctional family interactions began to impact the way I saw the world and relationships. This was also the 60s and the world was ablaze with change.

At fifteen, I was working after school at my parent's restaurant. I spent a lot of time with my father. He had alcoholic rages that shocked and frightened me. I became concerned and protective of him. He frequently drank and napped in his office, leaving me and the other waitresses to oversee the customers. I did not know it then, but the seeds of enabling were beginning to take root.

One afternoon, my Dad confronted me in the kitchen, his breath heavy with alcohol. He berated me over something that I did not understand. He was in a rage. I believed him when he said that it was my fault, whatever it was, and I take responsibility. I was terribly frightened and confused. I was rationalizing dysfunctional behavior. Was I responsible? Then I felt panic. My father's rage was inappropriate. I was unwittingly developing viewpoints, personality traits, and characteristics that were a dysfunctional way of interacting and would play a major role in the onset of panic, anxiety, and agoraphobia.

What did I do when my distraught mother, while holding my baby brother Mark in her arms, confronted my father over his drinking and irrational behavior? Why, I defended and protected him, of course! Guilt, shame, over responsibility, defending, protecting, denying, the true reality of situations and circumstances, and the people that I love, or think I love, became a daily occurrence.

When daily interactions are so confusing, it becomes easy to fall into an existence of keeping up appearances. This eventually catches up with you. At some point in our lives the appearances will come tumbling down. And then we have to face the music and deal with it. It is imperative to be true to our selves for our emotional balance and well being. But, what did I know about all of that then?

At eighteen, I moved to the Cape for the summer with four other girls. We were wild and carefree. I was young and in love with a much older man. He was handsome and worldly to my inexperienced eyes. I spent a glorious summer on his fishing boat, reveling in the happiness of the moment, and experiencing my first serious relationship. We spent time on the ocean at the helm of his boat with the wind whipping through our hair. I was delirious and in love. He was a heavy drinker and became unreasonable and abusive at times. This did not discourage me. I was in familiar territory.

At nineteen I worked as a cocktail waitress in Killington, Vermont. I was living with three other people in a beautiful ski chalet for the winter season. I was learning to ski with the young men that I met. They would wrap their arms around me and we would maneuver carefully down the ski slope. I thought I knew so much, and I foolishly thought I was so mature. I was full of pride and superficial illusion when my roommate told me that I attract men like moths to a flame with my mini skirts and long blonde hair. We smoked an occasional joint, drank wine and beer until dawn, and had bon fires in the snow. Life could not get better than this!

I navigated my way through new friendships and love interest while living on my own. I became friends with the bartender. One afternoon he allowed me to borrow his new El Dorado station wagon. I was neither afraid of the snow covered mountain roads, or the fact that I did not yet have my driver's license. I did not pay attention to these things, even though I should have. It was beginning to be very slippery as I careened down the mountain road totally oblivious to the danger. I attempted to make a turn on the bend in the road and continued straight off the side of the mountain.

By some miracle that I do not understand, the car landed sideways in a pile of snow covered brush. Another disaster averted in this careless life of mine. I managed to get out of the car, climb the hill, brush off my bruised but uninjured self, and hitch a ride back to the restaurant to break this sorry news to my very angry and unhappy friend. Oh well! Not to worry and life goes on. I was just relieved that I was not found out. Totally in denial about the ramifications of my actions my life style, or the events that occurred. Denial was becoming my friend!

At twenty-one, I have my whole life ahead of me, but my relationships, unknown to me at the time, continue to be with alcoholic men. I fall in love once again, we talk of marriage, and I believe that he will be the father of my children. When I become pregnant, he insists that I have an abortion. I am horrified and I feel betrayed. This becomes very perplexing and traumatic for me. My dreams with this man were not to be. It takes years for me to come to terms with such a loss.

At twenty three, I am rebounding from all these relationships that have broken my young heart and shattered my trust. It has colored my view of what a healthy partnership should be. I was becoming co-dependant on men that were alcoholics, although I was completely unaware of this at the time, because of course, we gravitate towards what is familiar.

With my self esteem and my sense of self turned upside down, I marry a man who is not only an alcoholic, but also, an addict. Why is that not a surprise? After suffering a miscarriage early in our marriage, I give birth to two sons that are the light of my life. We stay married for five unhappy, tumultuous years and then we divorce. Fast forward to a happier time.

It is now 1979 and I am the happiest I have ever been. Madly in love, two beautiful boys and it is my second wedding day. I am marrying into an Irish catholic family, with all the stuff that goes along with it. Dennis, my husband, is the best. I am just over the moon. He is a natural father to my boys and a hard worker. We settle into a new life together. We buy a house and I become pregnant with my third son. I am incredibly happy and in love. Then, my world starts to fall apart.

I am in the hospital in labor it has been 12 hours and my husband was asleep in the waiting room.

""Should I wake your husband? The nurse asks.
"Don't bother," I answer.

The trip to the hospital and the experience for both of us are not what I had hoped for. Alcohol had once again stolen a special moment. Heartbreaking! When I see this beautiful little bundle of joy, it is all forgotten! My husband, being an artist and photography enthusiast, chronicles our lives as a family in pictures from this day on and through the years. He captures some uncanny, amazing moments. They tell a story.

After giving birth to our son, I now had three children under five. Life became a struggle. My husband and I were arguing often over his frequent drinking and what I considered his harsh ways towards the children and myself. Looking back, I realize now that I was an enabler and had a lot of the dysfunctional ways of reacting, which created and exacerbated our differences. I cried and fought, and was very dramatic over things that probably were not so important. At the time, I thought it was heartbreaking and I was extremely emotional and self-righteous in who was right and who was wrong. I had the 'how could you treat me this way if you loved me?' attitude.

We had this crazy dysfunctional relationship. We loved passionately, we fought passionately. The kids didn't know what to think. We both grew up in alcoholic homes but didn't have a clue. We overlooked all the drama. I was into drama. We were a perfect match, very good at denial.

Early in our marriage my husband was involved with a business partner who lived next door to us. Together they owned rental properties. They would both drink and socialize frequently after work until things started getting a little crazy. He and his partner had come to a disagreement about the business holdings of some sort. There was a struggle for ownership and this partner began to threaten our family.

One night we woke up to the sound of breaking glass. 'What on earth is that?' we thought. We jumped out of bed and there was another sound of exploding glass. My husband rushed towards the sound, which was coming from our attached garage. He opened the door and was overwhelmed with a plume of black smoke. Our house was on fire! We both headed for the boys' rooms: he scooped up the two older boys and I ran for the baby's room. I remember how quickly the smoke filled the room as I pulled my baby to me and ran out the door. Dennis proceeded to try and put out the fire with a hose. There he was, standing in his underwear and trying to put out a house fire with a hose, while one of the neighbors called the fire department. God bless him!

It was a suspicious fire and no one was arrested. However, when the investigators came to talk to us later that evening, his business partner was standing in our kitchen acting concerned and surprised. He had, unknown to us, put a gun in our kitchen cabinet. What was up with that? Scary, frightening events started to build in my life as a result of dysfunctional people and relationships.

My husband rebuilt the house; we sold it quickly and moved to a different neighborhood away from his partner. My husband continued to drink and we continued to argue because of it.

One sunny day, when the baby was about 11 months old, I began to feel like I was outside of my body. Nothing felt right. My balance was off, and I trembled at the slightest stressful thought. I felt out of control, thinking 'perhaps if I take a walk,' 'perhaps if I take a nap,' or 'perhaps if I go shopping.' In the days to come, these feelings would come and go. I would attempt to go grocery shopping only to panic and leave the cart mid-aisle. I would drive the car a few blocks, become terrified, and have to turn around. I was always afraid, but of what? I never knew. I tried everything that I could think of to

13

calm myself to no avail. The panic increased with every week that went by. I did not feel safe.

"I need a break," I told my husband one morning. I felt like I was having a nervous breakdown. Maybe I was experiencing post-partum depression. Maybe I was exhausted from having three small children under five. Maybe all of this fighting and stress was taking a toll on me and I needed some rest. At this point I knew I needed some help because my panic was growing. I worried about something terrible happening to my children. I obsessed on my health. You name it, I worried about it. It became impossible for me to venture out of the house. I felt like I was going to collapse. So I retreated and stayed home, where I felt safe. The world just seemed like a very frightening place to me when I was outside of familiar surroundings. I felt like I was suffocating. I could not breathe.

I was such a perfectionist. The house always had to be in order. God forbid that anything was out of place! I did not want my little guys to be disruptive or unruly. I tried my best to keep order and peacefulness in my life of course; this is impossible when you have three active, healthy boys. What was I thinking?

One day, I had put all three boys down for a nap. I needed some rest from the commotion. I had just settled into a deep sleep. I hear a slight sound of business in the kitchen, and the undeniable laughter and giggles of my little guys.

"What on earth are you doing?" I scream.
"We wanted to surprise you with a picnic, mommy," they all sheepishly say, with peanut butter and jelly dripping from their fingers, and smeared over my nice clean cabinets and kitchen floor.

Well, that was it. I had just finished cleaning my house so it sparkled and I did not want anything to tarnish it. I was not able to enjoy the spontaneity of the moment. I was so wrapped up in my own issues of control and perfectionism. They had to endure my anger over something that was so innocent to them. How sad is that? If I could turn back time, I would embrace those moments with such joy.

Many times, I was unreasonable with my discipline, passing on the same attitudes and ways of dealing that I knew as a child. One evening, the boys would not settle down. They were excited and rambunctious, tossing pillows and wrestling. I warned them to sit still or there would be no Disney Special for them. The poor kids had waited weeks for this very special program.

"Okay, that's it!" I said, and off to bed they went: kicking, screaming, and crying. I would not relent. I was going to let them know that I meant business! If only I knew then what I know now. I would be so present in the moment of enjoying my children and the excitement. They were just children and they were excited. What a special moment of happiness with them that I missed. They did not know how desperately I was trying to keep myself together. I had not yet worked out my own pain, so I was blindly and arrogantly passing it on.

In the early years, the boys were subjected to arguing and inconsistency between my husband and I that must have been very frightening and confusing to them. Evan, my youngest son, would often disappear into his room and escape into vigorously riding his rocking horse. While doing this, he would cover his head with a box! That should have told us something. The poor little guy was doing his best to escape the commotion, noise, and craziness in our household. I was trying to keep my mind off the paralyzing fear and the physical symptoms that I was experiencing by keeping my house and children in order. I was at my wits' end.

I would like to think that in the later years of my recovery, that I did approach them, and their lives, with much more balance and joy. I hope that I have expressed in my actions and words, to each one of my boys, what a gift that they have been to me. I see their beauty as individuals and I hope they see mine.

I truly hope that they see the world as a parent, with different eyes than I did at their age. I hope that because of what we went through together, they now have a better appreciation for life and for me. I am extremely proud of them and love them with all my heart.

During this time, I continued to take care of my children, my home, and myself. I showered and dressed daily. I cleaned and cooked, but it was becoming increasingly harder to manage. I could manage inside, but I would panic outside. I tried walking down the street only to panic if I got too far. Cooking became a real chore. Soon my husband was doing all the cooking, driving, and the shopping. While I took care of the children and the house, and tried to figure out what was going on with my world and myself. Why was this happening? I was afraid that I had cancer or a brain tumor or worse, was losing my mind.

One day, I opened the phone book and searched for a counseling center. But how would I pay for it? We were struggling as it was. I found a counseling center, panicking as I made the call. At this point I was so desperate for help that I would have done anything to change what I was experiencing.

"How can I help you?" the voice on the line said.
"I need to talk to someone because I am having terrible panic attacks," I answered.

"Well let me take your name and number, and I will have someone get back to you," the voice said.

The waiting was the worst. Finally, a few days later, a very pleasant young man returned my phone call and I made arrangements to meet with him at the office He told me that the fee was according to our income on a sliding scale. Phew! That made it a possibility; we did not have insurance and finances were very tight.

My husband agreed to take me to my first session and watch the kids. Jeff was a bit younger than me. He was not the type that I pictured as a therapist. He seemed a bit off beat, but he was great at getting to the heart of things. As our sessions increased over time, I started to notice that every time I would be discussing what was going on in my relationship, or with the kids, or the anxiety that I was feeling, he would always stop me and ask, "So what was your husband doing while this was going on?"

"Oh, he was having a beer," I would answer.
"Hmmm," he would say and we would continue with our session.

I spent several weeks of counseling sessions rehashing my anxiety issues and what was going on in our family and relationships. One day, after listening to me and saying one of his many 'hmms,' my therapist looked at me, rubbed his beard and said, "I think your husband is an alcoholic."

To which I replied: "Oh no, he is not an alcoholic. He only drinks beer!"

Well, I needed to absorb the accuracy of this information. What is alcoholism? How does one define who is and who isn't? What defines dysfunction and being emotionally unavailable? Why does it create such instability and problems? Why does this create anxiety disorders? What is the cause? What is an enabler? How can I change this?

I read up on the disease of alcoholism, family history, how ones drinking impacts the other members of a family. How we can be affected from parents and grandparents, and generations of dysfunctional thinking and behavior. All of it a result of ones drinking or addiction that impacts the way a person thinks, and sees the world, others, and circumstances. How sometimes the spouse or children of an alcoholic gets even sicker than the alcoholic, emotionally, physically, and spiritually. Often there is an incredible amount of craziness that goes on in an alcoholic home. We spent a lot of time trying to make things seem normal, picking up the pieces from all of the insanity (a lot of which we created ourselves) until it finally caught up with us. Sometimes its not so crazy; it's subtler.

I was referred to 12 step programs, Al-Anon, and others, and researched literature. I began to read a lot on addictions and self help. I started reading an array of religious and spiritual books. This was a reflective time for me. I was very grateful that I was learning and becoming more aware of things that I could change in my life, to look at from a different perspective. At least there was a reason that I felt so out of sorts, so perhaps I could change things.

Maybe it was not physical after all. Maybe it really is a result of our environment and the people around us, and the emotional impact of stress and how one lives their life. Maybe, we really are affected by the people around us, and how they live their lives, the things they say, do, and the way we are treated. The way we treat others truly makes a difference in our wellbeing.

Later, when my husband did have insurance coverage, I heard about a treatment center at Spofford Hall in New Hampshire that happens to have a program for the spouses of alcoholics. I called and arranged with a neighbor friend of mine to watch the children. My husband agreed to drive me. Nervous and terrified, I was deposited at the door of the treatment center without much of a goodbye. I entered with trepidation.

It was an amazing educational and insightful experience to have. I took part in group and individual sessions, with all the emotional baggage that we all bring to this type of recovery program. One day after a particularly grueling therapy session, I looked at my councilor and said, "you know this place is like a life lab with a bunch of rats."

She looked at me with a glint in her eye and replied, "Exactly!" As if to say 'now you're getting it.'

I saw some of the most intense and raw emotions played out right in front of me. Suddenly I did not feel so excluded from the norm. It is bazaar and fascinating to see, and to hear how other people live, and look at the world, judge, and interact with others. But the most interesting thing of all, when I started to seek to be well and whole, I saw that we are not so different or crazy after all. Everyone else's life is just as crazy and no one else's life is a fairy tale. You realize that emotional needs in relationships are not met until one is in recovery. You cannot meet emotional needs of others until you are well and healthy. It is an awakening. Slowly, over time, I stopped blaming others.

I began to see how others have been affected and impacted by the people in their lives, and how I impact others. And miracle of miracles, I began to have compassion and understanding! I began to look at the world, myself, and my life with a whole different perception. Many of the things that I thought were *so* important became less so, and things that were not important became more so. I began to gain a perspective that I did not have before I cleared my heart and mind of all the nonsense. It is a long and winding road, this road to wellness. I was undoing a lifetime of dysfunctional programming. To change my thinking and view of my life history was a daunting process. It was the hardest struggle I would face.

I saw different doctors from time to time for my physical symptoms, still not convinced that the imbalance, the sweats, and panic, and irritable bowel was not reflective of a terrible disease that was not yet evident. Blood tests, x-rays, all types of medical work-ups. One doctor prescribed Valium. I took it for a week and felt more confused and anxious then before. 'No psycho-tropics for me, that's it! I will do this naturally,' I thought. I researched herbs and biorhythm, changed my diet (no caffeine, additives, or chocolate). I found all types of cures and suggestions to balance my health. Some worked and others didn't. In the end, our bodies are always healing and we need to research and find out what works best for our own wellbeing. I embarked on education collectively about health, addictions, and spirituality. I was hungry for answers and truth.

My journey began into the world of, among other things, understanding addiction and anxiety and its destructiveness. I soldiered on and the kids got older. With every year that went by I missed a little more of their childhood. I was so wrapped up with trying to function and understand addiction and my own anxiety. My husband was loving and supportive at times and at others controlling and insensitive. We were on a merry-go-round in our relationship and neither one of us understood it. I admire and respect his ability to be committed and provide for his family. We both tried hard to work this through.

It was difficult for me to go to school functions for the boys, sports, or social events. Often my husband went alone. He was a good father to the boys. The times that I would go, I thought I was going to die from the anxiety. It was overwhelming. I managed to get through, but I never enjoyed anything that I tried to do. Sadly, through these years, I was very self-absorbed and missed some of my children's best young years. It really is a very selfish time in one's life, but you could not have convinced me then that I was being selfish. I thought I was sacrificing so much. How could that be selfish?

The Beginning

I remember looking out the window one afternoon; feeling the warmth of the sun on my face and watching the children play with such gaiety and abandon. I felt such a sense of isolation and sadness at the inability to share in the joys of their childhood. All three of the boys, would go on to try their hand at different sports and school plays.

Often, I would not be there to share in their accomplishments. At times, I would push myself, but it always proved to be so exhausting, still fighting the fear. I was not yet aware of the techniques to be able to desensitize, not yet aware of the benefits of acceptance and letting go of all the things that were holding me hostage to this terrible dilemma.

I had an array of physical symptoms that were never ending. I was continually visiting the emergency room or a doctor's office, terrified that I was having a heart attack, or some god awful something! I prayed fervently please God let me be okay and please God let my children be okay. I always feared for their health and their safety. I just knew something terrible was going to happen. Often, this was not apparent to my family or others, because I kept these doom and gloom thoughts to myself, suffering in silence. The silence only accentuated my overall panic. The negative self-talk is very dangerous. With it, you can spiral very quickly into the depths of fear. We spiral down into fear when we do not neutralize it with hopeful or positive thinking. To get out of the place of confusion and negativity you must talk the feelings through with others.

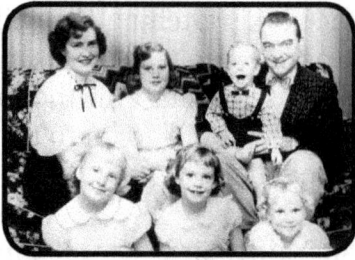

The Reed Family

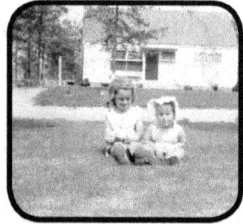

Denise and
Author

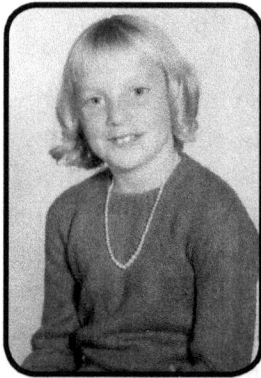

First Grade

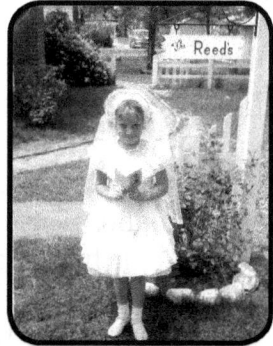

First Communion

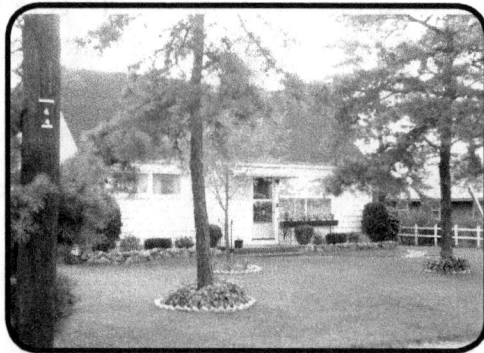

62 Bacon Road

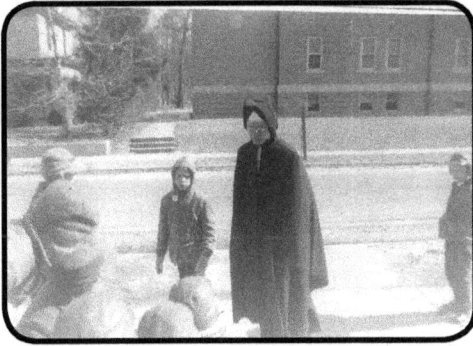

Our Lady of The Sacred Heart

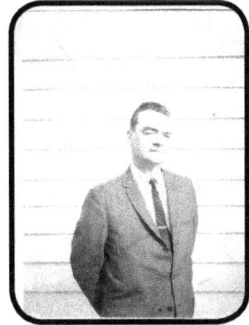

Author's Father

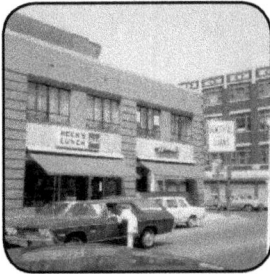

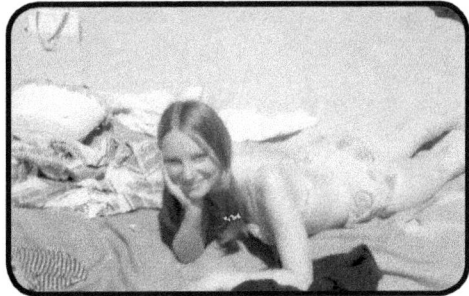

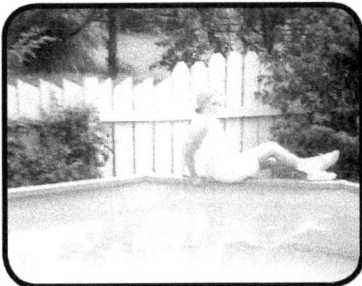

"The soul would have no rainbow, had the eyes no tears"

~John Vance Cheney

It's Okay

It's OK to be afraid of the things we do not understand
It's OK to feel anxious when things aren't working our way.

~Laine Parsons

I once heard it said that depression is really a very selfish place to be. When we are depressed, it is total self-absorption and anger turned inward. It is grief. Grieving for the life we are losing or the happiness that we have not attained. It is a paradox, because we also have to be kind to ourselves and know that whatever we have to do to get to the other side of this, its OK.

I was beginning to search religiously for answers, not yet understanding the difference between religion and spirituality. My mother and I attended a healing seminar at Oral Roberts University (ORU). This gave me hope and strength, for a while. I believed in the power of prayer, but I was not getting answers to my questions about life.

Amazingly, I still managed to function through those early years of anxiety. I do not know how, but I did. I even got to the point where I felt I was recovering enough to hold a part time job as a receptionist down the street at a dentist office. I could walk, but only those two blocks, and not walk any further. I would do certain things, but not others. This would produce a feeling of being safe in a controlled way, such as venturing out to the grocery, but only if my husband was with me. Another was going to church with the family, but only to sit in the back and leave early. I would only go to certain social events, not others, always fighting the fatigue that the anxiety would create. It was exhausting! I was always covering the fear.

Fear enveloped me constantly. I was never in a relaxed state when out in the public. I never knew when a full-blown panic attack would hit. It was so insidious and unpredictable. Depending on the day, I could sometimes do things and other times these same things, I just could not handle. I never knew when it would hit. I began to plan my life and my days around only what felt safe.

Christmas Eve 1988: *The tree is lit, the presents are wrapped, the children are sleeping. I am settling into an evening of reflection. I am thinking of how much I love my husband and children and our beautiful home. It was a good day. Then, for some reason, we started our stuff. I'm angry, he's angry. I'm pushing and he's shoving. I fall against the dresser and it falls against the window, shattering it. Dennis injures his shoulder and the reality hits us: this is getting dangerous! We stop. We hug and love each other with a sense of urgency. We are sorrowful and tender with one another. The window is repaired and morning comes. All is forgotten. Merry Christmas! We are the happy family once again. This is very confusing. With love, all things are possible. It was too painful to see.*

My husband and I got the idea that moving to the mountains in Vermont might be just what we needed and the kids needed: good, healthy country living. The stress of living in a city, the gangs in the schools, and our family dynamics would seem far behind. 'Let's make a move and find utopia!' we thought. So, off we went to the hills of Vermont. My husband was in the home improvement business at this point, so buying, renovating, and building was part of our background. We had just renovated a lovely historical home in Massachusetts. We sold it the first day that it was on the market, and within a month had packed up the kids and the house. Vermont, here we come!

I functioned much better when I was moving toward what I perceived as a new beginning or a change in my life. The move gave me hope. I understand that some people with anxiety and panic do not like any change at all.

For some reason, I was able to function in circumstances that gave me an escape from the reality of my situation. It was not easy, but I managed, always, battling that underlying panic and fear. I so desperately wanted things to change and was willing to fight the fear. Years later, when I really got completely well, I understood that it was the fighting the fear that kept me stuck, but more on that later. I had begun to unravel the mystery of looking inside of myself and my life and trying to become centered and balanced. I had a bit of treatment and therapy under my belt, but still had a long way to go.

We found ten acres of land in a beautiful village in Danville, Vermont. So what did we decide to do? We decided to build a bed and breakfast. Perfect! What could be better for someone who does not like to leave their home? What a great idea! Not really, but at the time it seemed ingenious. This also fit in with my idea of living a dream. The ultimate escape!

The move to Vermont and the building project that ensued was a wonderful adventure for all of us. The kids loved their new experiences in the country. The schools were such a welcome change. The air was cleaner and the stress was abating. My husband had begun to look at his alcoholism and Irish temper, and I was looking at my part in all of this. We read up on family dysfunction and the generational effects. Dennis began to get back to his painting. He was, and still is a talented artist. He stopped drinking, and was happy working in his element of building and construction. I was happy in my world of design, decorating, and planning.

The Inn came to fruition. I decorated the house with satin drapes and oriental rugs. I furnished the interior with antiques that I found at used furniture stores. I would labor over the cleaning and refinishing of old pieces, and delight in bringing them back to life. I strategically placed my husband's art pieces throughout the Inn, complimenting what turned out to be a very unique and eclectic décor. It was a comfortable, simple elegance.

We were meeting new people and venturing out socially. All seemed right in my world, but there were still the relationship issues: we were still fighting and making up passionately. Neither of us had really dealt emotionally with any of the past, and I still had that underlying anxiety.

We continued to live in a world of keeping up appearances. I was living a lie. On the outside, I wanted to look like the happy family with the loving husband but inside, of our home was often full of turmoil and inconsistency. One day I was madly in love and everything was great, and the next I was trying to make sense of the craziness that surrounded my family and myself.

The poor kids had a lot of mixed messages during those years. Through it all, I tried to be loving and attentive. There were times that I would have liked to have been more emotionally available and less overwhelmed. I would like to think I was a good Mom to my boys. A lot was kept from them. It was hard work to overcome the blocks and be there for them. I was sensitive to their happiness and loved them deeply. Why was life becoming so hard? What was this passive aggressive thing with my husband and I? Where are stability, calmness, and consistency? Alcoholism continued to have a rippling effect on our lives, even when there was no drinking. Until we began to address the anger and the hurt, and look at the reality of our lives with honesty and humility, we did not begin the road to true recovery.

We opened the Inn and continued to run it for three years. We had guests from all over the country and the world. It proved to be a very rewarding experience. We entertained the village residents with an open house and periodically hosted meetings for the Bed and Breakfast Association of the North East Kingdom.

Occasionally there were a few embarrassing moments when we could not hide our dysfunction. One time in particular, I had booked a couple from Tennessee. Everything was in order and we were preparing for their arrival. It was a quiet time of year. We mostly had seasonal guests, so we were closed in the winter. This was late fall and, at the time, we had no other guests.

On this particular day my husband and I got into one of our many heated discussions over who-knows-what. I was absolutely spent. The couple arrives and, of course, I am unable to greet them with my red and swollen eyes. As I was not in the best condition to meet them, my husband took care of the check in. We continued our discussion upstairs and I tried to keep my sobbing under control. This went on into the evening, and I was thinking I would never be able to do the breakfast routine. I was totally out of sorts. On and on it went.

You know, when you desperately try to cover up anything it usually blows up in your face. No matter how quiet I thought our expletives were, evidently we were not so quiet. At about 5:00 am in the morning we heard the start up of a car ignition. We looked out the window, and in the distance was a red convertible winding down our long driveway. Our guests were hightailing it out of there. No waiting for breakfast for them! Another blatant experience as to how out of control my life was becoming. Crazy times!

Trying to do something to change my circumstances, I read several biographies and autobiographies of others who had struggled with similar issues. I read a ton of self-help books during this period in time. They helped me gain lots of insight and education on relationships, alcoholic up bringings, different religious beliefs, and other topics. I was still trying to understand what my life had become. 'What is it all about anyway?' I would think. 'Why am I plagued with this anxiety thing?'

I tried meditation, exercise, diet restrictions, breathing exercises, self help groups, and therapy. One book that was extremely helpful to me was *Mental Health Through Will Training* by Abraham Low, a very insightful book into the physical symptoms of stress and anxiety. This book was written in 1950s and it is now difficult to find, however it is very beneficial in understanding panic, anxiety, and how differently people react to stress. It discusses the debilitating affects of anxiety and how to counter the physical symptoms by changing our thinking. This was a breakthrough for me. *It is a matter of how we think.*

My children did well. As they became teenagers, we went through the usual challenges of their growing years. My husband built another five homes on the land that we bought and sub-divided. One day I was entertaining a guest who commented on the Inns décor and said to me: "You really have a gift for decorating. Did you ever think of becoming a designer?" A light bulb moment!

I researched different schools of design and proceeded to throw myself into a correspondence course through Sheffield school of design. Another creative opportunity that wouldn't take me outside of my home. I could do it on the computer and through the mail. Brilliant!

It was 1989 and my whole world revolved around my husband, home and kids. I took great pride in appearances. Of course, nothing was as it appeared to be, and this was a major stressor. I continued in striving to keep up appearances. I would help Dennis design the houses, Dennis would build them. I was in awe of his talents. He always amazed me. I would sometimes work with my husband on the construction, as long as I did not have to go very far outside of my safe zone.

In 1992, after building several homes in Vermont and running the Inn for three years, we decided to go home to Massachusetts to see family and friends for Thanksgiving. Traveling was always difficult, but if I was in one of my better places emotionally from time to time, I would push myself.

This was not an easy feat, as there were still a lot of unresolved issues surrounding family, siblings, brothers, sisters, in laws, and ex husbands. Not a lot of happy memories. But, after enough therapy and self help reading, I was beginning to feel forgiveness towards the people in my life that I felt had hurt me. I was proud of my husband's sobriety and resilience and loved so many things about him. I was coming to terms with a lot of our history and my family dysfunction.

I was beginning to have compassion and understand that it was not all about me. Understanding the origins of family dysfunction, I was able to distance myself from the guilt and the confusion. The distancing was enough for me to realize that my family was just as affected in their own way. I saw them differently without assigning myself blame. Suddenly, I was beginning to have some self-esteem.

As we are driving back to Vermont after the holiday, the car radio was tuned to the news. The announcer said that the Caledonia Bank in Caledonia County had failed. This is the bank that we did business with and it was carrying our construction loans. This was a disaster!

This was during the savings and loan crisis of the 1990s and the country was in a recession. We knew that things were not great in real estate, as we had several spec homes that were not selling, but we certainly did not expect this! I was shocked.

"What will we do?" I ask my husband. We continue our long drive in silence.

Now my anxiety levels really began to rise. Everything we built and worked towards was unraveling fast. I started to feel really off balance once again. I went to bed for months, we did not plan for a spring opening of the Inn, we had no idea where this was going, and it became impossible for me to function. My world was collapsing, my dreams were crumbling, my relationship with my husband was intense, my children were demanding and at very vulnerable ages. I no longer had an escape or hope.

That spring we closed up our dream home, our beautiful Inn in Vermont. We eventually sold the remaining spec houses and the Inn for a big loss, then packed up a truck with our belongings and drove to South Burlington, where my husband found work in property management. We paid the rent on a small, crowded apartment for six months in advance with money still left in the bank. We had to figure out our finances. After a lot of financial wrangling, we worked out a deal with the banks and creditors. We were left with nothing. All of our savings and investments were depleted. We had lost everything.

It took an incredible amount of energy and effort to pack and move. Every day was a struggle, I felt totally exhausted. My world was in tilt: sound was distorted, and my balance was off constantly. I could not see clearly, I could not focus long enough to read a few pages in a book. Forget about even walking to the end of the driveway to get the mail. I could not do it. There were times that I was so exhausted I was almost afraid to go to sleep, fearing I would not wake. Somehow, with the effort of my husband and boys, we eventually managed to make the move.

Although I was proud of the fact that we did not go bankrupt and we had satisfied our financial obligations, we were devastated. It was difficult for the boys as well. That same year, my father was diagnosed with lung cancer. He succumbed to the disease six months later after a valiant fight through the chemo and radiation.

I am at peace with the fact that because I was in the beginning stages of understanding alcoholism and had been able to make amends with my Dad and heal past hurts. It was sad when he died I could not attend his funeral, because of being overwhelmed and exhausted from the events of that year. My panic and anxiety were full blown, along with feelings of despondence and depression. All these life and love conflicts that pierce the heart and the soul are held in our bodies until we acknowledge the truth of them. We may erase them from our mind, but the emotional impact will surface when we least expect it.

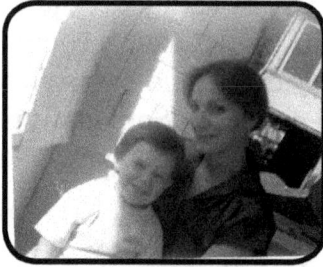

Evan and me

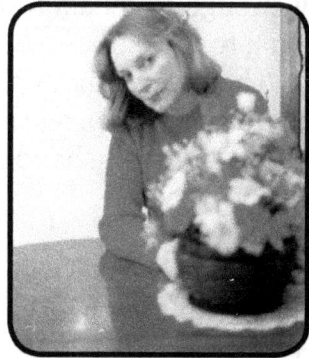

Truly, the eyes are the
window to our soul.

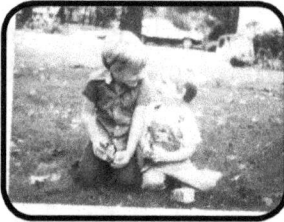

Justin and Todd,
Justin's first day of school.

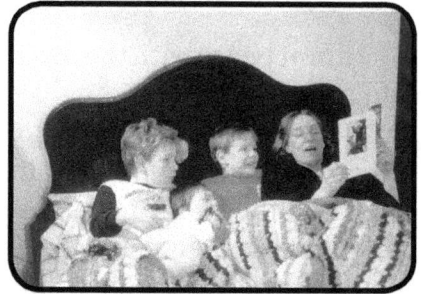

Always fighting
depression, and in bed.

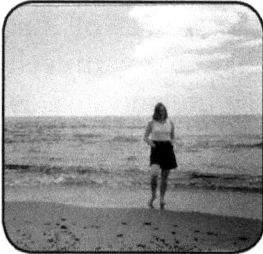

Contemplating dilemma
and trying to relax

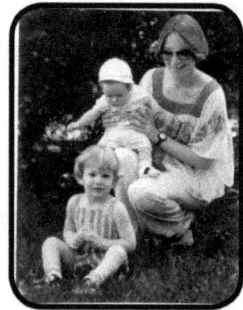

Evergreen Inn we built in
Danville, Vermont

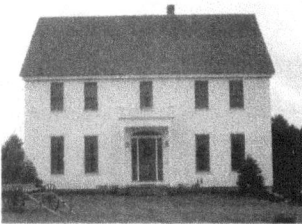

My Beautiful Boys Jus-
tin and Todd, before the
depression 1977

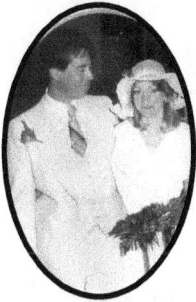

Dennis and me on
our Wedding Day

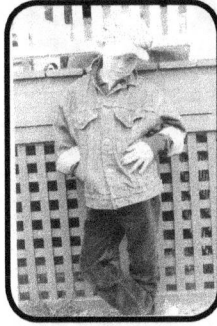

Evan striking a pose

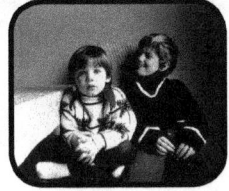

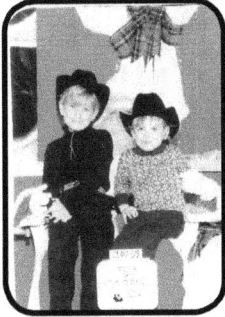

Christmas

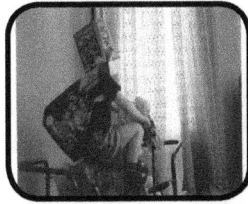

Evan escaping
the turmoil

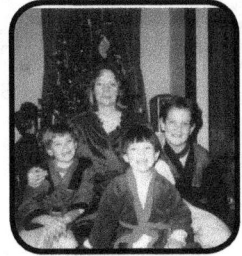

Not so happy
Christmas 1986

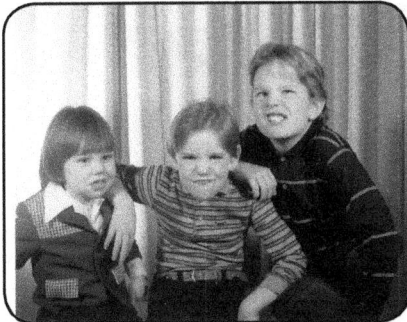

3 rambunctious boys

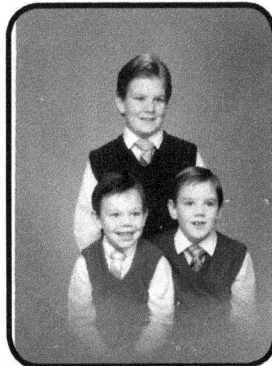

My Three Boys

"Sadness and emptiness are difficult to bear, but that which brings us sadness had once brought us joy."

~Flavia

There Was No Escape.

In the depths of depression, I could not even find comfort in my home, which used to be safe. My home, which had given me a sense of feeling somewhat normal, now became a prison. It felt like I was a prisoner in my own body. Often thoughts like "If I could only sleep forever..." went through my mind.

Sleep was my only source of peace, and even then at times my mind and body would race. It got to the point where I was lying still for eight hours, eyes fluttering, not getting one hour of sound sleep. It was a living nightmare. It seemed to have no end or sense about it. Sheer desperation and panic were my whole existence.

Earlier, when the children were young, the baby would cry and it would sound as if I was in a drum. The cabinets would close in around me as everything echoed. Sound was distorted and my senses were heightened. As thoughts raced, it felt as if everything was spinning, including me. Riding in the car, the sensation was uncomfortable. It felt like I was hallucinating with the distortion in sound and movement. I asked myself,

"Am I imagining this?" Everything seemed so surreal! It enveloped me like a giant black cloud. This began a cycle of feeding fear-into-fear.

Driving created terror, the very thought producing a weakness. The physical symptoms were very real: it was stress playing havoc. At times, my senses would play cruel tricks. Taste, smell, and sights were all distorted and definitely not functioning properly. Paranoia struck at full force. Keenly aware of my bodily functions, all feelings were magnified. Hearing my heart beat, my limbs would go numb, losing complete feeling. I describe it as being in a slow motion time warp. This fear would come out of nowhere and I would panic!

These sensations would come and go. I would begin to feel normal, and then another sensation would obsess me. I was literally obsessed for hours with each new symptom. I stayed in the clutches of terror for months at a time. I would feel as if there was a bed of marshmallows under my feet. It felt like the ground was caving in beneath me. When I mentioned this to others, of course, they would look at me strangely, who could relate to that? Is there anyone who has experienced any of this? This was not talked about. I had no idea what I was experiencing or why. In effect, I was having a complete breakdown.

Fighting this desperately, with every fiber of my being, my body was so tense that I created exactly what I feared. I retreated and stayed home where I felt safe. The ridiculous expectation and fantasy of what life should be was literally making me sick. I was setting myself up for failure. My fantasy was one of the perfect life as the perfect wife and mother, with the perfect husband, and, of course, the perfect children. How ridiculous! Then, I would have weeks and months where I functioned somewhat normal, whatever that was.

At times the experiences of panic and fear were joined by a

feeling that was like walking in a fog. Feeling detached from my body. Sound and sight were distorted. My world was in tilt. "What is happening to me?" I silently cried. These episodes would come and go, striking without warning.

Later, when I could manage to get my strength to venture out, I found massage and breathing exercises very helpful in relaxation. For a time, I hired a massage therapist to come to my home. I started taking vitamins and drinking herbal tea.

When we begin to understand the physiology of our reactions to danger, the fight-or-flight response, we realize its connection to our physical symptoms and our unconscious reactions to stress, which in the case of anxiety and panic is usually a result of conflict or ambivalence in our lives and our relationships. These things need to be resolved emotionally, by facing the fear and the truth of our lives in the past and present. We need to break through our own denial. Pro-active therapy (desensitizing) and constructive talk therapy is extremely beneficial to making progress. It is a long process to recovery, but worth the work to get to the other side.

After about six months of not leaving my apartment because I felt absolute terror when I did, I began to experience severe vertigo. I could not walk without feeling very weak. I did not have the strength to get out of bed. This I knew was something that needed attention. I made an appointment with an ear doctor thinking maybe this was the cause of my anxiety. He diagnosed me with mennieres disease. Now, I have a very interesting theory about this diagnosis: I did a lot of research and came to the conclusion that an inner ear imbalance can just as easily be a result of stress, as it can by physical or environmental causes.

Mennieres is caused by a build up of fluid in the inner ear. The causes are environmental, from chemicals, damage to the vestibular nerve by an injury, or a diet high in salt, caffeine, additives, or nitrates. I believe this build up of fluid can also be caused by stress. When you think of how you hold your jaw when tense, it seems very possible that this fluid could get caught in the ear canal when we are anxious.

I stopped drinking coffee, caffeine, high salt, and foods with nitrates or additives. One of the big additives is aspartame. Aspartame is used as a sweetener and preservative. It is horrible for our body and some people have allergic reactions to it. It should not even be on the market, but it still is. It's even in chewable vitamins! We think we are getting a healthy vitamin and it has this awful ingredient.

All additives, food dyes, nitrates, and MSG are things to be aware of, especially if we have a sensitive constitution. Research has shown that most people with depression, anxiety, addictions, or numerous physical ailments can often be attributed to food sensitivities or allergies, to mold, or to environmental toxins such as pesticides or chemicals. Medicines, even though a doctor prescribes them, can be very dangerous and toxic to some of us.

When we are under severe stress, our bodies cannot metabolize what would otherwise be okay. It plays havoc with our well being when we are in a heightened state of fight or flight. I believe stress and anxiety is responsible for a majority of inner ear symptoms and afflictions. I went organic and treated headaches with cayenne pepper. I ate bananas for the potassium that is depleted from stress, and started drinking bottled water and herbal tea (decaf). I was trying to rid my body of chemicals and anything that would cause sensitivity.

After years of trying to keep a lid on the panic and anxiety, I was now completely housebound and agoraphobic. I tried to change everything that I could to combat this. Eating healthier, dealing with my issues from the past and present. I studied different religions and lifestyles to try to find answers. I quit smoking. I got involved in born-again Christian philosophies. I prayed and accepted Christ into my heart. This made sense to me. I questioned my Catholic upbringing and the conflicting Christian teachings of the church.

I studied further, researching personal experiences by Christian authors, looking for answers. I listened to Christian tapes. I listened to TV evangelists. I read up on the life of Christ. I studied biblical teachings. I got all fired up in the fervor of the "born-again experience." I did this for sometime. Prayer became very important to me, and I experienced what I believed to be little miracles in my life. I was growing spiritually and becoming stronger and healthier.

Then I had more life questions. Some of the religious teachings no longer made sense to me. I was still struggling and it did not seem that my prayers were being answered. Alot of the Christian teachings do not make sense to me. Some do and some don't. I begin to question Catholicism and Christianity, thinking: "There must be more answers to this cycle of life. Why do some people have so much, and others so little? What is the purpose?"

"Why do some people go through life so healthy, and others so infirm? Why are some people so rich and others so poor, and struggle so? Why are some people blessed with such beauty and others not? Why do some of us leave this world so young, and others so old?"

I do not believe that God or a higher power is so unkind. I believe that behind all the teachings and confusion there has to be goodness somewhere. I began to study A Course In Miracles. I read up on the mysteries of the pyramids and crop circles, of Tesla and St. Germain. On and on, I researched. My belief system turned upside down.

In the years before my depression, many things pointed in

that direction. I came to know and understand things that, in the years before my depression, I had yet to see. Before, I battled overwhelming anxiety attacks and agoraphobia. I was totally unaware of it, but as it happened, I had no choice but to search for a way to get well. In my desperation, I would have done anything to change what was happening. I was isolated and housebound for years. I sought every available source of information and every avenue of cure. I researched, reviewed, and debated information that was available. I found a wealth of knowledge and information that is indisputable.

Many of us have been misinformed concerning religion, spirituality, and sexuality. Consequently, bitterness can become a way of life that destroys our very being. Our spirits are in rebellion as to what is truth. I have come to understand that it is essential that these thoughts and feelings surface and be understood. It is necessary for emotional wellbeing and true happiness.

When we become open to growth emotionally and spiritually, our lives take on a dimension that we never thought possible. We begin to know the meaning of serenity, and being at peace with God, ourselves, and the world around us.

I have a memory at 18, walking the beach on the bay at Cape Cod, wondering who God was, and if indeed there was a God, how he managed to be so indifferent. There was something, a power greater than myself. I felt desolate, alone, unimportant, and disappointed in the Supreme Being that was called God. It was the Vietnam era and I wondered, as did other young people of my generation, how could God allow war, poverty, starvation? Why were some healthy and others crippled?

Why did young children die so young at the hands of psychopathic killers or abusive parents? Why? Why? The questions seemed endless, and for every answer there was another question. I looked out over the ocean that beautiful

May day-the water was a rippling blue, the wind on my face felt wonderful, the smell of the air was breathtaking. I looked at the beautiful world before me, and knew that there must be answers, but what were they? It was the beginning of a conscious spiritual quest.

My spiritual sensitivity began to develop this particular summer. It was to mark the beginning of my seeking and growing in a very sincere way: But, little did I know what the years ahead had in store for me, and what experiences, lessons, and sadness that would bring me to my knees.

"'And what is as important as knowledge?' asked the mind; 'Caring and seeing with the heart,' answered the soul."

~ John Vance Cheney

Seeking Truth

Healing from a Christian Perspective:
Notes from my journal, 1980s

As I see it: alcoholism, or any obsession, be it drugs sex, or gambling, whatever the case is an addiction because of emotional starvation and emotional starvation is a result of distorted interaction in ones life, which is really a spiritual sickness or more appropriately termed a "disconnect"

We often have distorted ideas and viewpoints: When we look around at all the people who are lost, unhappy, or addicted are they searching for some sense of belonging and acceptance? The bottom line is we cannot do it without a connection to God. He is our source, in all things. Our spirits need that connection.

I have begun to research the bible as a means of understanding: It seems that I want to devour this book on an intellectual level and feel it in my heart and spirit There are some scriptures that speak to me:

In Philippians: 8 verse, Ch 4: Paul tells us about positive thinking, pure thinking , hopeful thinking. He says, "finally brethren, whatsoever things are pure, loving, and just think on these things. This is important. Think on these things," he tells us. He reminds us of the absolute importance of hopeful thinking!

Luke 4-18: Set free at liberty those who are bruised.

Romans 12-2: We are our past! Another scripture tells us, but be ye transformed by the renewing of your minds.

John 3-15: Jesus said, "come to me all ye that labor and are heavy burdened. For I am the way , the truth, and the light, and the truth shall set you free."

Revelations: Very interesting: Christ will return to set up his kingdom for 1000 years. What? I find this fascinating and curious this last book of the bible.

Lots of controversy and misunderstandings-misinterpretations: Religious, spiritual, denominations, different churches, spirits, spiritualists, demonic, occult, satanic, angels all of these areas are interpreted differently. It depends on what source of information from authors, evangelists and others.

Ephesians 6-11 6-12: For you are not wrestling with flesh, but of principalities of darkness of the unseen world.

Matthew 11-29-30: Jesus said: "Take my yoke upon you, and learn of me. For I am meek and lowly in heart: and ye shall find rest unto your souls. For my yoke is easy and my burden is light." Let none of us then regard our defects as incurable!

Simple truths: Sanctify means to purify. Sin is a Greek word and it means simply to miss the mark. Repent means to change our ways or take a different path. Most bondage in our minds comes from auto-suggestion, it is not real! It is not the truth.

Testament means will, as in legal document.
Old testament dealing with God the father.
New testament dealing with God the son Christ.

Jesus had brothers and sisters, according to some writings. All different.

Before the days of Noah: it never rained, the world was encased in a protective bubble, and when the great flood came it was the protective surrounding about the earth rupturing, as a result of mans separation not a punishment is one evangelist's interpretation.

Great men of the bible:o had there trials and tribulations: Elijah by the juniper tree cried "God take me I want to die." The scriptures tell us in Hebrews chapter 11 that Elijah was close to suicide. In any event, he was despondent. He experienced many trials emotionally. he needed deliverance. Paul was frequently speaking of the thorn in his side, in any event they had trials David, Jonah, and Job , Abraham in Genesis, Jeremiah, king Saul, many struggled with depression and despondency.

The bible is a very symbolic book: There are many dual references. This is important to remember in discussing things in scripture.

The bible was written over a period of 100 yrs for the New Testament and thousands of years for the Old Testament to be written beginning with moses to the time of Christ. And then after his death the books of Mathew, Mark, Luke, and John were written. They were businessmen, doctors, scholars, and lawyers. Right down to revelations. God was directing the work of the bible through these men, but, they are human.

Beware of the man that stands on the street corner with his head bowed and hands folded as if in prayer, for I will say to him when the time comes "I never Knew you" Jesus referring to false believers.

Greater is he that is in you, than he that is in the world: When God be before you who can be against you? He will give you the desires of your heart... for he will open the windows of heaven and pour out his blessings upon you.

These are all quotes from scriptures and they sustain me. Immersed in understanding this mystery, studying, and praying I want to know truth! I am convinced that my answers are all right in this book of the bible as confusing as it can be sometimes and the more I study, the more confounded I become with some of the ministers that are preaching.

I often pray and repeat the scripture, "Be still and Know that I am God."

"Be still and know that I am God" this calms me. I really believe that when we reach out to God with the sincerity of our hearts, God will reveal himself to us right where we are. Somehow, and someway, we will know his presence in our lives. We are all on a different walk and on a different path. We all experience God in our own unique way.

I believe that it is important to research different philosophies and religions and to expand our understanding of life and spirituality. We need to know what it is we truly believe, otherwise how do we know what our convictions are. Christians believe the messiah has come. The Jewish faith is still waiting. Why the discrepancy?

If we have not experienced sadness, how do we appreciate Joy? Would it be any good otherwise? As my heart is weeping, my mind and spirit are seeking. I will continue my searching until with every fiber of my being the true purpose of my life is revealed! I feel a lot of discomfort with the contradictions in the Christian teachings. There has to be answers that make sense! I do not believe that this is the only answer. I think there is more. I begin to study further, A Course in Miracles.

Starting to research outside the realm of Religion I absorb all that is possible. Taking in information and expanding my understanding on all different levels. It seems as if I cannot get enough of this knowledge that is out there in the world and the universe. There is so much to learn! So much more than just what religions teach us. I am aware that many people stay in bondage in their minds because of religious teachings. This perhaps is one of the reasons that people struggle with panic and anxiety. They do not know their truth, they do not know their purpose in life!

I begin to understand all of these different spiritual beliefs and teachings. Different religions, different philosophies all have something to offer. I understand that they all work together on some level. Maybe one teaching or one religion is not the only truth. I begin to believe that there is more to understanding our life and our purpose, once we are removed from the limitations of prejudice and dogma. I believe in Jesus, but I also know that there is more to understand! Spiritually, metaphysically, philosophically, cosmically all seem to blend. The Indian prophet Sai Baba, the Islamic, and the Hindus all had prophets that performed miracles. Edgar Cayce from Virginia Beach, he diagnosed diseases and cures while in trance all new and interesting!

"Seek and ye shall find," I believe in Christ, this I know in my heart is real and true. There have been many prophets, Buddha, Krishna to name a few. I also, know that the spiritual realm is very mysterious and that the universe is calling to me. It is beckoning with an abundance of knowledge and wisdom "simple truths". I am humbled in my quest for answers and how little at this point that I really "know" about God, and this life of mine, and the world that we live in. What about physics, and the Egyptian Pyramids, and Astrology and perhaps life on other planets. Are there other worlds out there? I begin to search and to read and to search. Who is God really? Who is our creator? What is our purpose? What is our truth? What is myth and what is reality and are there many realities?

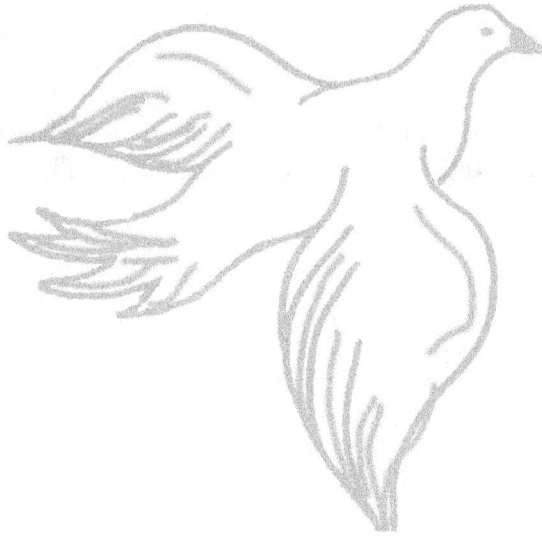

"Let none then regard these defects as incurable. For God will give you the grace to overcome them!"

~Eileen White

This Thing Called You

I begin to have big questions, questioning everything that had been taught to me as a child and into adult life, about my religion and my catholic background. There is a power greater than ours, but I also believe there is more to spirituality than is understood at this point. Some spiritual philosophies suggest that our life is an illusion that we create so, unconsciously we write the script! This is completely foreign to my belief system. I begin to research further for understanding and truth.

Ten years of my life have now been spent battling anxiety and panic attacks. Some years were more difficult than others. I am not leaving my house at all, I have not driven a car in years and the agoraphobia is full blown. I again pick up the phone and make a call, only this time I need someone to come to me, it would not be possible for me to go to the office.

I call a random number and ask the receptionist if they have any counselors that would be willing to make a home visit, "oh we do not do that," she says.

"Please ask, I am terrified to leave my apartment I need someone to come here." Why cant you leave she says? Because I am terrified that I will collapse I tell her. Well can your husband bring you to the office? NO, I SHOUT! I apologize, and do not want him involved.

I am aware enough at this point to know that I am so angry with my husband that a lot of my emotions and conflicts are all wrapped up in this crazy relationship and life of ours. I am cognizant enough to know that he is not completely to blame, that I am responsible for a majority of the issues that I am dealing
with, but I still do not know how to separate what is reasonable and what is not as far as my anger.

Feeling completely let down in my aspirations in life, and unfairly blaming him. If he was more loving and attentive; if he made more money; if he did not have such a volatile temper; if he was kinder; if he hadn't been an alcoholic our life would have been so much better; whine, whine, whine. I wonder what he was thinking!

He must have had lots of complaints of his own. It couldn't have been easy for him either.

A few days later a call comes from the agency, she has someone who is willing to make a home visit and would like to interview me. Thank you God! We set a time and meet a few days later. To my surprise he was just a kid, not much older than my oldest son. Oh boy, what can he possibly know about anxiety. He's a student at the university and studying for his degree in psychology.

After an initial intake of information he says to me, so what is it that you are most afraid of? I tell him everything. He asks questions about my husband, past, children, and the family alcoholism. He says, "I think that you have an anxiety disorder and that you are agoraphobic." "Oh no, I do not have any disorder. I just need someone to talk things through with." Let's see he says, "panic attacks afraid to leave the house, and has been struggling long term. What would you call it?"

I would call it being burned out from all the stress in my life. Like having alcoholic husbands, and growing up in an alcoholic home, two marriages a divorce, dealing with dysfunctional ex husbands, houses burning down, crazy business partners, moving umpteen times, losing a business and dream home and everything you own to a financial crisis. Struggling to survive and having three kids to raise in a crazy household. You know like post-traumatic stress syndrome or something, don't you think? Can we do this without labels or drugs?

I have another theory about all this psychological labeling that the medical profession seems to be so keen on. This to me is the worst thing that anyone can say to someone who has anxiety, to label him or her with a disorder. It is just one more thing to worry and stress over. To tell them they have a disorder of any kind, or to cover symptoms with drugs is ridiculous! What is it about that the medical profession does not understand? Why do they promote all these drugs for anxiety? Instead, of proactive talk therapy and diet and lifestyle changes?

I believe the drugs inhibit our recovery. Perhaps, temporarily, while one is at the height of their struggle and is unable to function. Even under these circumstances, I believe it is often best to be drug free, but with an understanding of what is happening, and the origins of where it all comes from. We must begin to change our thinking, perspective and how we view things. Our bodies follow our minds and our thoughts. This is how we begin to recover. The feelings of anxiety and panic abate after our thoughts and thinking are healed. It is a long and difficult process and the best gift that we could ever give to ourselves. So, we need to be patient with recovery and ourselves.

Most often one just needs to relax, get centered, change their lifestyle, diet, and surroundings if possible, and their thinking. Begin a journey of recovery with a supportive and balanced therapist. Reeducating our thinking and talking through a lifetime of issues with someone that we trust is an amazingly therapeutic tool.

To be able to let go of the past and its hold that it has on us. It is not easy. It is a journey of discovery about ones self. And trust is a big issue because it seems to us that our trust has been betrayed so often in our lives.

I continued my home sessions and began to make progress. Steve worked with me every week faithfully. I began to walk farther each time we met. We started leaving my house block by block. And as we walked and talked, I vented, and he gave me feedback. Regardless of how much I panicked we went a little further each time, my therapist was kind, but firm. You will not die Sharon, I am right here, he would say, what is the worst that could happen? He would ask. I learned to turn what ifs into so what!

We talked about my upbringing and my family, and how I never felt close to my parents or any of my brothers or sisters. At this time in my life, I perceived my family as very judgmental, non-accepting, very opinionated, and non supportive. We talked about my dating years and sexual experiences, and we talked about my first love when I was 18 with a man who was 42. We talked of the guilt I had over having an abortion at 20 and the betrayal that I felt from the man I was in love with.

We talked of my first marriage and my ex husbands addictions, and the affairs- and how I thought that the miscarriage that I suffered was a punishment from God, or the universe, or my karma, or whatever. And then we talked of my divorce. We talked of my second alcoholic marriage and how it affected me and my children, and that I had a part in

56

this that I needed to look at, I was a classic enabler. Oh great another label!

We talked of the conflicts, ambivalence, and anger. Of my children and how blessed I felt to be their mother. Of the guilt felt in not being able to have the energy to be present for them and their happiness at times because of the depression and anxiety. Wishing I could turn back time, knowing what I know today. They were beautiful healthy boys and I loved them dearly. There was much interior conflict and feelings of being overwhelmed with obligations and worry. We talked of alcoholism and addictions, its origins, and its affects. We talked of my fears, and my panic and the physical symptoms as well as my fear of driving.

We talked of my view of the world, and perfectionism that seemed to have a hold on me. I talked about my parents and being the middle of seven children and feeling lost in the shuffle growing up. Working at my parent's restaurant and my father's drunken rages. We talked of my carefree days during high school and the trust that was broken with friends and boyfriends, because I was such a people pleaser! The summer that I worked at the cape, and the crazy experiences that I had. The winter that I worked at a ski area, the first time living on my own.

We talked of all the aspirations that I had when I was young that I never attained. During and after high school I worked in nursing homes as a licensed CNA with hopes of becoming an RN. I loved to sing, I loved to dance, why did I not pursue any of these things?

We talked of how when one is affected by any type of addiction that they treat others with disrespect through their words and actions. Learning that I need to take responsibility for my part in this as well, perhaps, I need to look at my own personality defects and family dysfunction. Of course, this I did not like to hear.

Low self esteem is created when dealing in a dysfunctional and emotionally abusive environment and how skewed our world becomes. We look at things with judgment rather than acceptance. I talked and talked and talked and then I cried and cried and cried, for what seemed like forever. We continued my therapy like this for 6 months and I made a lot of progress during this time. And then my therapist changed the game.

One bright sunny day I notice I am looking forward to my morning session with anticipation rather than dread. I am beginning to feel better and stronger. There is more calmness and less anxiety. There are feelings of hope again.

There is a knock on the door, Steve my therapist enters and says to me, "I think we should try to take a drive, what do you think?" Terror strikes full force. NO WAY! I scream, I am not driving! Tell me exactly what it is you feel when I mention driving he says. I feel total panic and like I would have no control. I feel like I would collapse at the wheel, because I feel so weak from panic when driving.

I explain to him that it is not driving a car that creates the fear but, the feeling of weakness that overcomes me that terrifies me. Because then I have no control and feel like I will collapse and die. I am not afraid to drive, but afraid of the weakness that is felt when driving, do you understand? And somehow in the recesses of my mind, I know that this represents so much more, but I do not yet know what.

The following week in one of our sessions I ask, is there a support group for people who are recovering from anxiety and agoraphobia? He looks at me, with a slight smile, and says, yes, but no one ever shows up. I laugh, the humor that he was alluding to, did not escape me.

My world is beginning to expand beyond my home once again. I am more comfortable out in the open and around people. Steve and I venture into stores and public places for short periods to begin with and then at longer intervals. Still nervous and apprehensive I agree to try driving fighting the fear, and moving through it. I remember something from a mental health article on Will Training "do not feed fear-into-fear" It is the fear of the fear that is holding me back. So let go and go with it. Stop fighting it.

One morning Steve says to me, I would like you to drive me to the corner. Go as far as you feel comfortable, we can turn around when ever you want, Reluctantly I agree. Angry with him, but I proceed to drive. As I am driving to the corner, he asks me to tell him on a scale of one to ten what my anxiety level is. For weeks we do this and I tell him it is at a level 10. Every time I reach the corner I begin to sob and don't know why. Feelings of sadness and grief while experiencing a weird feeling of abandonment over come me.

One day there is an amazing breakthrough. Talking, while driving, about all my feelings, fears, anger, and sadness there is a moment of clarity. With tears streaming down my face, I understood the significance of my agoraphobia. I was so angry with my husband and our marriage, as I understood it at that time, I was afraid of leaving him. This anxiety was masking all the things I did not want to look at in my life. The inability to drive was keeping me from leaving! I wanted to stay, and leave. It was a paradox. I was ambivalent and conflicted, I loved him desperately! There was so much mental confusion.

A very old memory was brought up; I was just six years old and sitting behind the stage at a dance recital waiting with excitement to be called out on stage. My sister Denise does her tap dance and I do ballet. At the end of the recital, we are waiting with all the other dancers to be called out individually to receive our flowers from our families.

The anticipation and excitement for me, as a six year old

is palpable. They call my sisters name, she takes a bow and receives her bouquet, after all the other names are called, I am sure that I will be next, but my name is never called. Instead, they call my sister again and she takes another bow and receives another bouquet.

The curtain closes, the lights go down and I am sitting alone. I am devastated and I am sobbing uncontrollably. This moment freezes in time in my six-year-old mind. As I am describing this memory to my therapist, I am crying as if it was happening to me in the now. I am astounded and embarrassed at the force of my grief over something that happened to me as a child. How is that possible to have such an impact on recall 40 years later? Our rational minds tell us this is ridiculous and yet here I was grieving over an incident that my adult mind would have excused as ridiculous. Excused because I understood that no one was to blame, these things happen in life, it was not intentional, and as my mother explained the florist had made a mistake.

I felt so much freer and totally released from that memory once I dealt with it with honesty and allowed myself to feel and cry about it, even as an adult after all these years. Today, I truly have no feeling about that experience, isn't that interesting? Imagine the impact on children and adults that are intentionally emotionally, physically, or sexually abused. This is where all of our Psychological problems come from.

I believe it is important to do what ever we can to respond to situations regarding loved ones and others who are emotionally traumatizing in the moment. If we are emotionally healthy ourselves, we are more attuned and, we take steps to limit the emotional charge of incidents such as this.

For example: I would like to think that as a parent I would try to rectify a situation such as this by responding with love and compassion and finding a way to let that little girl feel important in a moment that was unintentionally missed.

Today, if I were the mother of that little girl, I would realize the importance of the moment. I would have discreetly gone to the announcer as quickly as possible and explained the error. So my little girl could take her bow, receive her flowers, and be acknowledged. My mom bless her heart, just looked at me and said, well, now dry yours tears, we will go have ice cream. She missed the whole point for me. The different awareness then when my children were small makes me wish I had done so many things differently.

I missed those moments in my children's lives as well, and often missed the point with them. And so it goes from generation to generation. Until, someone hopefully, breaks the cycle of dysfunction and insensitivity. Wellness and clarity is such a gift!

The truth is things happen all the time in life that are not fair but maybe we could nurture one another a little bit differently through our lessons in life, with compassion, kindness, and insightfulness.

I no longer feel sadness for that six year old it is just an experience, it has no emotional charge. Well this is what happens with our lives continually. As our child and adult self it is imperative that we deal honestly with our emotions in the now. In this way, we can release the impact, so it does not have a hold on us. If it remains emotionally charged, it will screw up our thinking and our feelings, because that is the core of dysfunction. We need to cry, scream, and laugh, in the now. We must do whatever it takes to be well, whole, and honest with others and our self. We have the right to feel our feelings. Rather than be told it doesn't matter or it is not important. Or what's the matter with you?

It was an incredible lesson of how we are impacted with every fiber of our beings from the time we are born until we leave this earth. Our bodies hold our emotional experiences, and they are imprinted in our hearts, minds, and souls. We need to release the intentional and unintentional hurts that we are holding. We do that by being honest with others and our self through all of our experiences in life. At some point everything expresses itself in our life, either emotionally or physically. So, we really need to be clear and at peace. With how we are treated and how we treat others. What goes around comes around for sure!

Well, after this breakthrough, I must have cried for days. It felt as if I actually had experienced a death. I felt such grief and shame at my life. All of this anxiety and agoraphobia was an unconscious protection from running away from the people I loved. This was the beginning of the mystery to my struggles unfolding. What awareness! I felt like a lifetime of shame had been lifted after my 9 months of proactive therapy. I finally understood so many things all at once. All the talk therapy, research, reading, and healing was coming together for me.

Soon, I was driving miles, and then high ways. And before I knew it, I no longer had panic attacks at all. My energy levels increased. We continued this experiment for weeks until I was able to drive further and further.

Around this time, I learn of my Jewish ancestry of my grandparents on my mother's side. Why didn't you tell us I ask her? She looks at me incredulous and answers, your father's parents wanted me to embrace the Catholic religion and culture in order to marry into the family. It was different back then.

I didn't think it was important she says. Unfortunately, growing up we never knew our grandparents on my mother's side. Judgment and prejudice were passed on from generations to us. I am thinking of all the things in my life that are not as they appear to be. A veil of denial, on so many levels, surrounds the truth of my life. Keeping up appearances was beginning to feel very uncomfortable. There was denial in my life with my marriage, children, and family. This I knew was at the root of my anxiety.

And then I got angry and in order for me to right my world, I told everyone F ... you! I was not in a good place. But that did not last long because I realized that perhaps one could be honest with diplomacy, not always, there are times that it is, what it is. But for the most part I have learned that telling everyone what you think without choosing your words carefully is not wise. So I still needed a lot of recovery. I was very angry with a lot of people and about a lot of things in my life. I still needed to learn humility, surrender, and forgiveness.

I still needed to work on my life, issues, and self. I was a long way from understanding my history, and this journey. At this point, I start to become kinder and more accepting of myself. I am patient with my progress. I am recovering and emotionally healing. No longer, take on the guilt and shame; understand this does not have to be done perfectly. What a relief! I am becoming comfortable in my own skin.

I start to study and read eastern philosophies. Things begin to come together; questions make more sense to me. I really expand my understanding of life, reincarnation, past lives, Karma, near death experiences and theories on cosmic phenomena .You name it, I studied it, reading, and reading. After reading so many different points of view on life and religions, I started to read biographies. I begin to see with a different eye, and gained a new perception.

I had an insatiable need to understand what it is that creates dysfunction. I wanted to understand spiritually and the purpose of life. I came to believe that most struggles with panic and anxiety in our lives are a result of conflicts and ambivalence of any number of things. Often it is over ideas such as religion, sexuality, family, relationship issues, emotional, physical, verbal abuse, and addictions. Living up to what we think others demand or expect from us rather than living our truth can cause a great deal of anxiety.

We need to face and accept what we are denying. These things have an unconscious hold on our psyche. By facing it we accept, release, detach and reeducate our thinking. We cant change our past, but we can change how we think about and how we react. By using what I call proactive therapy, this is almost like aversion therapy where you are slowly exposed to the situation or reality that is creating the fear.

"My over promised self set free"   (John LaCarre)

Often our thinking and reactions are this ingrained from childhood and generational programming. Anxiety and panic means there is conflict somewhere in our thoughts and emotions. Biographies and autobiographies or memoirs are very helpful to us for this very reason. There is an undeniable real benefit to stepping into other people's experiences, in that you begin to get a perspective on life that may not be possible otherwise. I slowly started to notice an increase in my energy.

The problems lies in how we think about our lives, people, self, health, bodies, and especially relationships, they are a big one! We can change how we see and process reality. By changing how we see things we change how we feel, which then results in changing the way our bodies respond to our thoughts and feelings. And, it often has nothing to do with what you think you fear. In reality, this fear probably is masking the underlying real problem, which you don't want to see!

In addition to self-help and biographies, I expanded into the metaphysical and past life regression. I saw spiritual advisors and shamans. I separated what was beneficial to pursue and what was not. I wanted to explore all areas of life and different philosophies, and others experiences. I read a ton of memoirs and gained an incredible amount of insight.

What felt right and true to me I kept and what did not, I didn't keep. This is a twelve-step slogan "take what you want and leave the rest" a great philosophy. I wrote letters to some and let go of others.

I continue my counseling and twelve step programs. I go to meetings but not as frequent as others. Sometimes, I feel that the people in the meetings are just as judgmental as the outside world. It doesn't work for me on the level that it appears to work for others. I am not convinced that a lot of the people that I meet really understand panic and agoraphobia the way I experienced it, although I do know that others express understanding anxiety to different degrees.

I am more comfortable pursuing my recovery through philosophical and spiritual means. However, I absolutely think that 12 step programs are a valuable step in my healing. Somehow, I understand that I still need to interact with others in this capacity to get to the next level. So, I continue to work on my recovery and myself. I know it is important to be with people and all the discomfort that goes along with it. It is an imperative to face the fear. I am getting stronger.

I have worked very hard on my recovery emotionally, physically and spiritually.

With time and patience I make progress, I am coming in to my own, I am healing!

I decide to use my training as a CNA from years ago and apply for a live-in-home care position with an elderly couple, staying in their home Monday through Friday with weekends off. My children are teenagers in High school. Dennis is with them in the evenings he is a good father. It gives us time to reflect and regroup. We all benefit from this time apart. My husband and I read books by John Bradshaw Several of his books on family dysfunction and dynamics are enlightening. We also read an array of books on inspiration from authors with a different perspective.

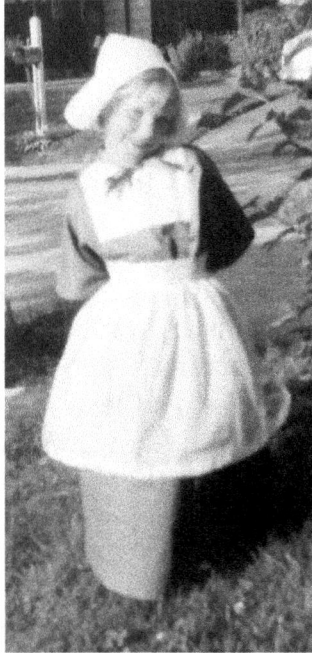

The never to be forgotten
Dance Recital

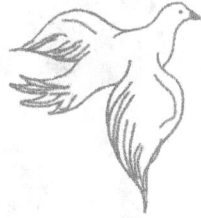

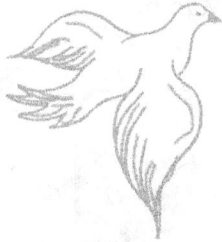

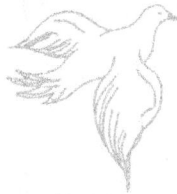

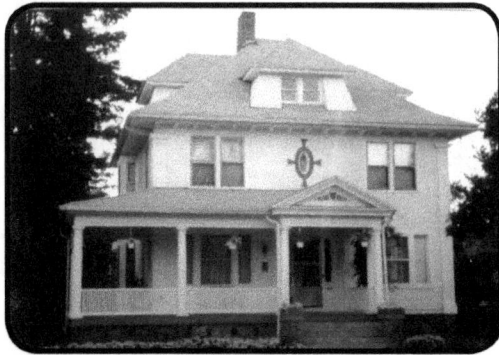

Historical home we renovated. built in
1901; 100 Marengo Park

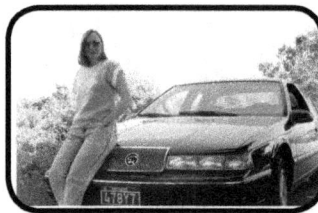

Debating a drive

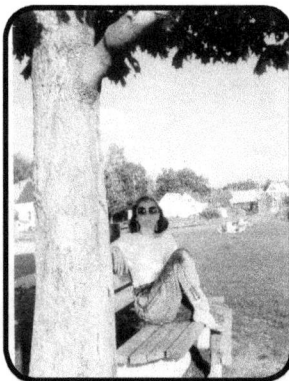

Reflecting

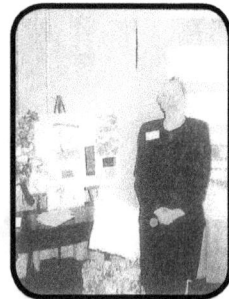

Showing
Apartments

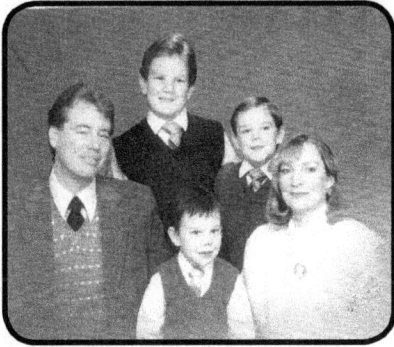

The McCarthy Family, Dennis, Justin, Todd, me, and Evan

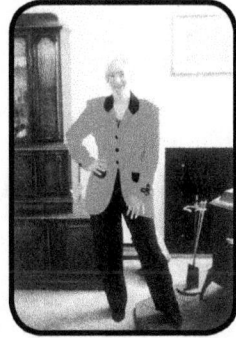

Ready to take on the world. Feeling very confident

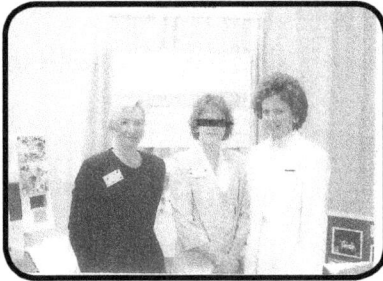

A Very Proud Moment

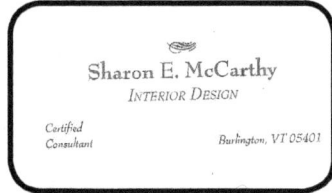

Sharon E. McCarthy
INTERIOR DESIGN
Certified
Consultant   Burlington, VT 05401

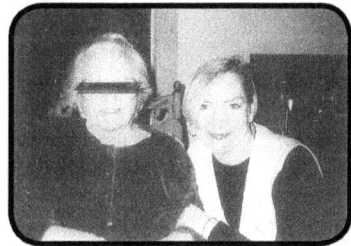

Assisted Living Client when I was a CNA

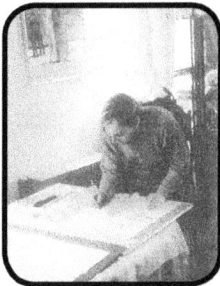

Assisted Living design project

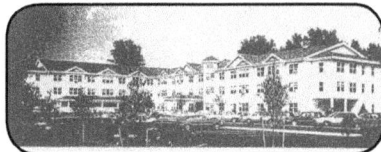

Never lose an opportunity of seeing anything that is beautiful,
For beauty is God's handwriting, a wayside sacrament.

~Ralph Waldo Emerson

Progress

I don't have to drive, although at this point I am beginning to drive again. This feels comfortable to me. I can handle this and have hope. Getting out of my surroundings, and contributing financially, what could be better? This is a beginning to me, it does not feel overwhelming it feels safe.

I work in this capacity for over a year. I am feeling better about my life, marriage, children, and myself. I had the time and space to reflect and sort things through. I am beginning to want more in my life and to participate in ways that had been impossible. I decide to take a class for a semester at Champlain College in Hospitality Supervision and Management.

This proves to be beneficial in more ways than one. It is necessary to interact with other students, many younger and I have to face my fears, and give presentations. One morning I am scheduled to speak in class on my experience in running an Inn, Yikes! I remember that it is ok to fail and the important thing is that I try. Nervous and trembling I decide to brave through it.

At lunch walking through the cafeteria, I feel confident and there is a spring in my step. I have not felt this way in ages what a feeling, its liberating! That dark cloud is beginning to lift. My self-esteem increased with each fear faced. I am beginning to realize that we all go through life, feeling that we do not quite fit in. I am beginning to think who cares! Another what if turned into so what!

I have now completed the hospitality course. This will be useful someday. I am anxious to get out and enjoy the world a bit, but how? Taking the class was an incredibly innovative way to desensitize my fear of people and public places. My anxiety decreased with each week. It was like learning to swim, or ride a bike. It took practice and persistence. I have come to a certain acceptance of my relationships with family, husbands, and children. I am no longer sad or angry.

By this time my oldest son Justin has graduated and is in college working on a degree in media communications. My two younger boys Todd and Evan are still in high school, and we begin to feel the rumblings of alcohol and drugs in their social circles. Oh that's just great! My husband and I have just begun to get our lives on track from the history of alcoholism and dysfunction, and now we have to confront the affects in our children from our past. But, of course this is the pattern, does it ever end?

We get into family therapy and address the issues surrounding our crazy lives. We cry, we scream, we laugh, and through tear filled hugs, we console one another and try to make sense of our journey together. There are many intense and angry fueled confrontations. I see the unfortunate evidence of my past fears and perfectionism taking hold in my children's lives. They are repeating of course, my patterns I inadvertently passed on. They continue their therapy.

My husband and I continue with our couples therapy and educational opportunities on family dynamics and addiction. We try to change the way we relate to each other and to the boys, we make progress and are encouraged.

A lot of blame and heartache comes to the surface. We try to move forward with some sense of understanding and love. We are connected whether we like it or not! We talk of our struggles and of our dreams. And I hope and pray that my children will come through this, and be in a much better place at a much younger age than I was, or my husband was to begin their recovery.

I hope against hope, that they will not have to endure as an adult, the struggles of unraveling a lifetime of dysfunction. I hope they are addressing it constructively and understanding dysfunction and addiction at a much younger age. I hope they are blessed with the openness to grow spiritually and emotionally through this. I hope with the right direction. Trusting they can put this part of their upbringing behind them and release the emotional charge of hurts and anger in their lives through talk therapy. Through self help awareness they will have a chance at a happy and productive life.

I hope that they will get it and not pass on all the nonsense and dysfunction to their children. That they will be patient, kind, and loving parents, because they will be emotionally present and balanced.

I pray that through our experience as their parents that we have broken the generational cycle of addictions and dysfunctions. I hope that they find it in their hearts, to deal with and forgive the past, and any hurt that I, or their father, or step father unwittingly caused when they were young.

I pray they will not become full blown alcoholics or addicts before seeing its destructiveness. I pray that they will have the desire for a better life. I know that alcoholism and addictions are the result of a spiritual void in our lives. I hope my children embark on their own spiritual journeys, for wellness and wholeness. Because they deserve the best that life has to offer. But, I also know, they have to walk their own walk. I think they have a good chance at it.

Hopefully as parents we lay the groundwork the rest is up to our children. I believe we were appointed to have this experience together, somewhere in the ethers, before we were even born. This I believe is the basis for our struggles. We are learning lessons together. We are one another's teachers. Somewhere in the heavens it was decided that we would take this journey. This makes sense to me. I have accepted my life as it is no longer feeling such ambivalence about my relationships, emotionally and spiritually, I begin to heal.

I am now at a place in my life where I want to step out in the world a bit and use my background in design. I apply for a position at a Furniture and design company in Burlington. On a beautiful fall day I walk in with my resume and ask to speak to the manager. He is not available, but the woman at the desk takes my resume and says she will have him call me. As I leave, I am sensing that this would be exciting and I could do this. I just do not know if I could keep my nervousness in check if actually offered a job.

A week later I am called in for an interview. I have such panic and anxiety about the prospect of the interview I almost call and cancel. Once again, I remember how far I have come and I must face the fear to get to the other side.

Regardless, of how uncomfortable in the moment I am aware that this too shall pass. However, I recognize the difference of realistic fear. I am OK.

I walk in to a fabulous quaint shop on Church Street, in the heart of Burlington. Chris, the owner, introduces himself and shakes my hand, we exchange pleasantries. I tell him that I am available from 11:00 to 4:00 in the afternoon, three to four days a week. The full day would be too much but this I do not express this to him.

I tell him I am certified in design and have a good eye for color. He asks me about the Inn that we built, and if I was good with people. Determined to be positive, and look forward not back, I reply, oh yes! After several follow up phone calls, which were very nerve racking, I was offered the position.

To my surprise, I felt nervous, but excited. I was trained on the desk routine, and then briefed on the origins of the oriental rugs. In my element, I just loved the environment of design and the people that I worked with. The family who owned the company was terrific and I felt very comfortable. I became very efficient at being able to talk to the customers about the furniture and the rugs, I was very good with customers, and in time became very confident. I was able to talk to customers about any subject. I attribute this to my insatiable reading of biographies and self-help. You name it I could relate!

Suddenly, I started noticing that while I was taking care of customers they would talk to me about all sorts of things that were going on in their lives. I was happy to listen, and maybe give a little bit of insight into what they were sharing. I also took interest in their décor and asked lots of questions to help them make decisions. I discovered that because of my design background I was very proficient at visualizing. Also, because of my experiences with anxiety and depression had made me very insightful, and compassionate.

Well this was a winning combination, because people are really lonely in their lives and they love to talk. And I was good at listening. With my background and knew about issues so I was very happy to talk and to listen. I felt like I hit the jackpot!

I would share things they could identify with.

I understand that we all have problems, and nothing any one says or does surprises me. I would listen and nod my head, and relate with willingness people felt and understood. People sensed that I truly was enjoying talking to them in the moment. They felt acceptance and I felt acceptance in return, how wonderful! I loved being with people, I loved sales, and I loved my job!

There are the usual challenges and competitiveness with one another among the other employees. I usually manage to maneuver through this with diplomacy and come out unscathed. I am once again learning how to deal with people and their emotions in the real world.

My years of therapy, and understanding of dysfunction becomes a huge asset in a sales environment. I don't take it personal or judge. I don't think that I am the problem. I understand we all bring different backgrounds to what we react to and I have a detachment that is invaluable. I look at my part in situations and I try to be flexible. This is new to me. This is great!

I went on to work full time, five days a week and to become one of the top sales people in the company. Customers increased and my sales increased. My husband and I started ballroom dance lessons. We started to socialize, and have dinner parties. I have good relationships with friends, co-workers, and my employers.

I am surrounding myself with only emotionally and spiritually balanced people. Life was good! I started to meet with clients as a designer. I did the design and decorating of two assisted living facilities in Burlington. The projects consisted of sketches and working up a layout from blue prints to the actual building.

This was an amazing accomplishment. It was a time for me to break into the business as a consultant. I used my training to do the layouts to scale from blueprints. I did all the purchasing and decorating. Once the building was completed, I did the ordering of window treatments and furniture placement. I promoted the assisted living at a senior fair. This was good for me personally, and for the company. It was a winning moment in my life. It was wonderful!

At this time, my husband was involved in creating a web site for his art. He became accomplished enough to start selling his work through different venues. He was invited to have quaint art shows at small cafes throughout Vermont. Eventually he sold pieces to collectors in Vermont, and New York. This was a promising beginning.

I am free of anxiety and panic for several years. I am accomplishing things in my life that I never thought possible, driving everywhere and anywhere. I have lots of energy and feeling good about myself. I cut my hair short and I love it! I am deep into fashion and love to get dressed for business and meet customers and clients. I have an enjoyable circle of friends and have come a long way. I am beginning to feel happiness and moments of real joy in my life. Wonder of wonders! I work for three years for this company. I appreciate this time in my life immensely and what I have accomplished.

"Life grows ever lovelier as each day comes and goes with happiness unfolding" like the petals of a rose.
Mary Ellen Lowe

My husband and I regrouped financially and we are once again, in a position to look into buying a home. We secure a mortgage for a cute little house in Burlington, not far from downtown Church Street, where I work. We renovate and move in. I enjoy the process of decorating and settling into a place we can call our own.
I am thrilled to be living in the downtown area, with all the

hustle and bustle of a city, how things change in life! By this time our middle son Todd had moved out and was aspiring to try his hand in the culinary arts and film. Our youngest son Evan was just graduating from high school.

Christmas of that year we entertained family and friends. We set up a fabulous tree adorned with sparkling ornaments and enjoyed a lovely cocktail party. At this point I understand that there are people who drink socially and it is not a problem for them, and there are people who don't drink at all, and probably should not. We accommodate both.

I am far enough along to be comfortable in either environment. My history no longer dictates how I approach my life. I enjoy people in the moment without putting any restrictions on them being much more accepting. That year we were more active with dinner parties, dancing, and social functions than ever before. We were having a ball!

In 1999, we decide to put together a resume with our collective experience and skills in hospitality, building, and design, perhaps we could find a position in estate management. We gather references from personal and business associates. We compile our accomplishments and experience, and notify an agency in New York. Private Estate Mgt positions offer potentially excellent salaries.

One evening we get a call from a woman in Palm Beach who is interested in interviewing us for a position. She speaks to Dennis and confirms that if everything checks out with our references and background check etc, we will schedule a flight for a personal interview. Terrific! This would be an interesting experience indeed!

Later that week we get clearance from the agency. We arranged to fly out the following week on a flight she has arranged and will pay for. Dennis and I both have vacation time from our jobs, we notify work that we will be gone for the weekend. We fly to Florida. I actually flew albeit a bit apprehensive. Once we were in the air, I started to enjoy the marvel of it all.

Landing at the airport and she sends a car for us. We meet with Mr. and Mrs. M. They have a lovely mansion in Palm Beach, overlooking the bay. After an initial interview and tour of their large estate, Mrs. M informs us that they are looking for a couple to run the household, would we be interested? Absolutely! We both say, with out missing a beat.

In Vermont, we give our notices to our respective employers. In two weeks, we say good-bye to all of our friends, and business associates, they all wish us well. We decide to rent the first floor in our house in Burlington to my two sons, at a minimal cost. In exchange they will take care of, and oversee the property for us. We create a small cozy apartment on the second floor, so that we have a place to stay when visiting. We pack up our car and drive for three days reaching our destination in Palm Beach.

We are thrilled with the excitement of the possibilities, and intrigued at the thought of being in Palm Beach with the rich and famous. We think the job responsibilities are something that we can handle. We are happy with our living quarters. We are getting familiar with the area and getting into a routine as we meet the other staff. We work hard at proving our competence and try to be very professional. We confer with one another and decide, we will run it like the Inn.

And then reality hits. Mrs. M. is familiarizing us with the different serving dishes in her silver cabinet, as she does a lot of entertaining and dinner parties are one of our major responsibilities. I ask her a question regarding the many dishes that she has just displayed. She looks at me with a look of disdain and says in a loud voice IS THERE A MEMORY

PROBLEM? I knew right then and there this was not going to work!

What on earth are we going to do? Now, I know that people are not perfect, and when you are faced with such rudeness, you hope against hope that, this is not par for the course, but you usually find that it is. And when you have had as much background and education in dysfunction, as I had, and you understand the origins and the red flags you are way ahead of the game.

It's kind of like fore warned is fore armed and boy had I been fore warned. I wanted nothing to do with this type of personality, especially since we were living and working in her home. I worked too long and too hard to get myself balanced from these types in my life. Forget about it!

Well, we muddled along through six weeks of rudeness and disrespect, trying to figure out, how to get out of this mess. All the while, I would whisper to Dennis " I can't STAND this or her!" It is like being held hostage when you feel that you have no choice, but to soldier on until a solution presents itself. My solution finally came, without any planning on my part, during one particularly stressful evening. We had given yet, another dinner party for eight people, without so much as a graceful thank you from Mrs. M. We are both exhausted and so discouraged. What a big let down this whole thing is, it was a nightmare.

The contractors had been working on a brick walk outside of the side entrance. After cleaning up in the kitchen after the dinner party, I proceeded down the brick walk to empty the trash.

Forgetting about the construction, stomping my feet with anger, frustration, and exhaustion, suddenly my foot slips between two bricks. Snap, I am on the ground writhing in pain, my foot is as limp as could be. Oh my God! What happened? Dennis screams. I think I broke my ankle.

Be careful what you pray for, you just might get it. I was definitely praying for a way out of this situation. I also believe that the universe gives us what we need, according to how we think and conduct ourselves. The expression that I was using the most while in Palm Beach was "I cant stand this" How interesting is that? That I break my ankle so I can no longer stand?

My body had physically followed my thoughts and words. I once read an article that described a theory about different physical ailments and symptoms that come about according to our thoughts and words. (i.e.) If a person is constantly saying "what a pain in the ..." the result is hemorrhoids. "I don't give a ...." the result is constipation. " I can't see straight," the result is vertigo or dizziness. " I am p...... off" the result is bladder infections. " I am just sick over this" or you make me sick, the result is stomachache. " I am worried sick" the result is stomach ulcers. "You are driving me crazy!" The result is emotional problems and turmoil. Everything in life is how we think, because it really is all an illusion.

If we are aware of all the terms and ways that we describe things it is no wonder that we are so afflicted. Cause and affect, we are what we think. Our thoughts are very powerful. During my experience with vertigo, I was constantly saying I am so angry that I can't see straight!

I am on the ground in excruciating pain waiting for the ambulance to arrive, when Godzilla (Mrs. M.) shoves a glass of water in my face and says "here takes this its an aspirin" no, no, I say. I will wait until I know what's going on. OK fine then suffer! She says, with indifference. I was definitely in pain, but I also knew that I was going to need surgery. And if I did have surgery, I didn't want to go under anesthesia, I would want a spinal.

I had read that if you even have one aspirin before surgery it could interact and cause complications if you have a spinal. It can cause internal bleeding. I waited 24 hours for the top orthopedic surgeon to arrive. Turns out it was a massive break, my entire left foot had snapped off at the ankle completely, and my ankle had been splintered into pieces. I found that if I held my foot in a certain position it was bearable.

After x-rays and blood work up, the nurses kept insisting that I let them shoot me up with pain meds, they kept coming into my room with the needles all set and ready to go. Please NO, I would say and they were amazed that I was willing to experience the pain. It was not excruciating unless I moved. So I tolerated it.

The medical profession is so used to people taking drugs for any thing and everything, that they cannot comprehend alternatives. It is unfortunate.

It was worth the wait. I had a wonderful orthopedic surgeon, and a wonderful anesthesiologist who both worked together to recreate my ankle. It was quite complex and they agreed that I could have a spinal, only if I had not had any meds not even aspirin they said. I was thrilled that I had stood my ground.

I had the surgery with a spinal, and they did give me something to quiet me. I woke up with such clarity, the doctors were impressed. I was impressed. I think there was such clarity, because I had no drugs, before or after.

I continued to be drug free during my convalescence as well. I think we push drugs for all kinds of things unnecessarily and consequently, the medical profession creates more problems and disease. Think about the onslaught to our bodies when trying to metabolize these chemicals and drugs. It is mind-boggling.

And that is just what psychotropic drugs do. They fog our brains and boggle our minds more often than not. If we tried to do things as naturally as possible., we would have much better results. And I believe that this is the case with drugs for depression and anxiety. I believe they inhibit full recovery and healing.

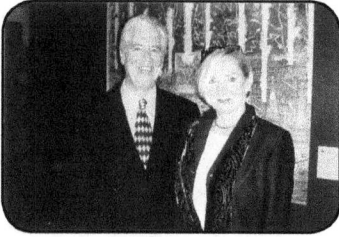

Estate Management
New York 2003

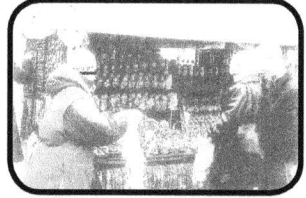

Russia 2004

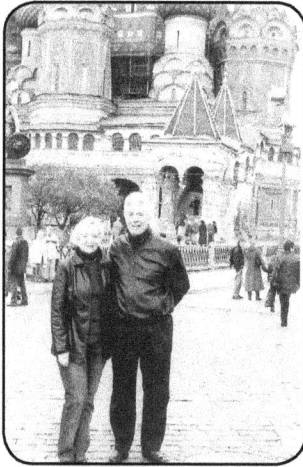

Lenin's Tomb

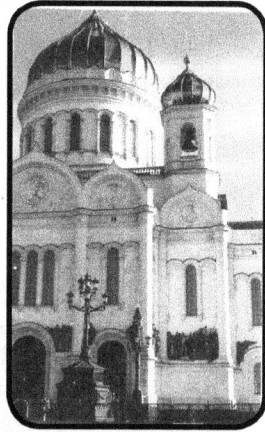

Red Square

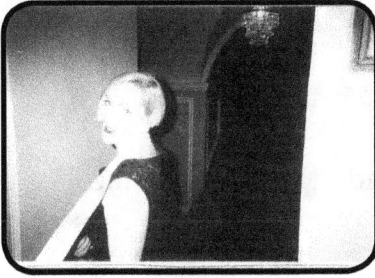

At The Russian Ballet

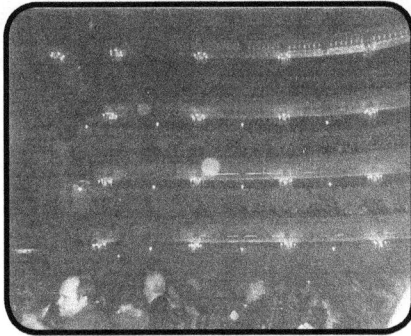

The many tiers of seats at the Ballet

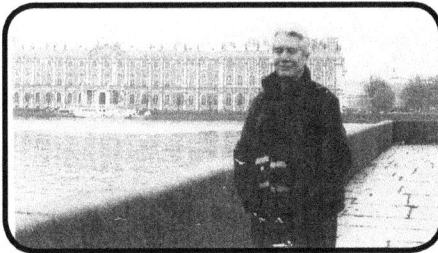

The Hermitage

Love begins at home, and it is not how much we do... but how much love we put in that action.

Mother Teresa

Going Home

We left Florida a week later. Our car trip back to Vermont was not uneventful. My leg in a cast, wobbling around on crutches, and sitting in the back seat of our car, my foot wedged between the bucket seats, to keep it elevated and extended.

We are driving down the highway at about 70 miles an hour and out of the blue, a metal ladder falls off of a construction truck right in front of us. It crashes to the ground, crash, bang, screech. We go right over the ladder. The cars in front, behind, and beside us are swerving out of our way.

This could not have been good for my foot, which had so delicately been put back together. We get out of the car grateful to have survived, my foot and ankle still in one piece. We discover, miraculously there was minimal damage to our car or my ankle. We are shaken, but alive! We continue with our road trip. I am worried about not getting enough calcium, and drink a lot of ensure. I could not wait to get home.

After three long days of travel, we pull into the driveway in Vermont. We get settled in and I begin my 6 to 9 month recovery and rehab. I call the insurance company because I believe that water therapy would be helpful in my healing.

After 6 weeks, I am told to start walking with my cast. This does not make sense to me. Would it not be more reasonable to walk in a pool with the resistance of the water? I ask my doctor sure, he says, but the insurance company will not pay for this kind of therapy.

I call the insurance company again and insist that this would be very beneficial. It does not make sense to put full force on a bone that is not yet healed. It will make it heal flat and wide. Well "I will look into this and see if there is something we can do," the secretary says.

The insurance company finally agrees to pay for water therapy at the Y. I can go and take rehab classes for 6 weeks. Great! I make progress. In my research, I find that it takes approximately 9 months for an injury to heal. Three months for the muscles and tendons, another three months for the nerves, and another three months for the bones to kneed together completely.

Now, how many people do you know who get right back on an injured limb? And then take an array of pain meds while trying to heal. Does this make sense? I believe that the refusal to allow the body to heal appropriately and the onslaught of pain medications really restricts the possibility of complete and whole wellness. I pampered my foot and ankle for nine months.

I did water therapy with resistance, because it is necessary to start to put pressure and work the muscles and the bone, to help kneed together and prevent atrophy. I believe that it is a mistake to place full force on a bone that is healing it needs a strong foundation first. The other thing that I took exception to was the removal of pins. I did not have the ninepins removed as suggested. I have left them in my ankle and had no use in further surgery. My foot and ankle healed beautifully.

I never have pain or discomfort. I can work long hours on my feet and dance without a problem! I attribute this to my efforts in being drug free through my surgery and healing, and water therapy, plus visualizing a completely healed foot as I was recovering. It is amazing how we take for granted our bodies, muscles, and our health. All the little things that we can do every day when our bodies are working right, but when we are out of commission and need help to do the littlest things for ourselves. To have that experience of infirmity and rely on others is frustrating and humbling. I prayed and tried to think positively.

That summer, after just getting back on my feet, we receive a call from an agency in Connecticut. They still had our resumes on file from the previous year. Would we be interested in a position on Long Island New York? Of course we would, we were completely amazed at the timing.

I had trust in my resilience and the experience of the last year had not shaken my faith in the overall goodness of others. I had learned a lot about interactions with others, and believed that together my husband and I had an amazing education and experience to bring to this type of career.

I knew that we had a lot to offer the right family, with the right situation. We were poised for success in the hospitality background and believed that there were incredible possibilities.

We agree to meet our future employer's assistant at the W Hotel in New York City the following week. We left Vermont on a scorching hot day in the middle of July. We were to meet for an interview in the hotel lobby. We were excited with anticipation at the possibility of a prospective job offer.

We meet with ML, who turns out to be the COO of our future boss company. He is high profile, based in Europe and has a summer home on Long Island. They are in the process of major building and renovation and need someone with a construction and hospitality background. They would like a couple to run their estate like an inn. They have a large extended family and need someone who understands the dynamics.

They were very impressed with our background and skills she says. How perfect is that? Dennis skills in building and construction, my skills in design, and collectively our experience in hospitality and all of our efforts at understanding family dynamics will come together for us, finally!

In September of 2000, we get the final offer for the position. They would like us to start in a month. Once again, we make arrangements with our house in Vermont. We pack, say our good byes to family and friends, and embark on a journey that is uncertain at best.

It is always a balancing act working in this type of environment. It is imperative that it be a good fit, not only with skills and experience also with personalities, understanding family dynamics, and life style. These components all come into play in the initial probationary period, for the employer, and employee alike.

Efficiency, loyalty, honesty, and confidentiality are first and foremost. We were pleased to be working in this capacity. It was a testimony to our abilities and our integrity. And we found that with all the different family dynamics, we were good at negotiating all different challenges, regardless of what we were presented with.

We were honored to be working for them. They were a large extended, loving, active, and enthusiastic family. They were usually respectful and appreciative. We were given the authority and freedom to run things the way we saw fit. We initially ran just the household. After a time, we were responsible for hiring and training the staff.

I became the family's assistant, responsible for itineraries, and the families schedule and children's lessons, etc. We both took care of the financial responsibilities. Dennis negotiated with contractors and vendors, landscapers, pool companies. We did the entertaining, either arranging for catering or preparing the dinner parties ourselves. Eventually we became very adept at preparing and setting up for large buffet style entertaining in the cabana.

We would also personally put on formal sit down dinner parties for up to 8-10. We did all the shopping, errands, driving, cooking, scheduling, and overseeing a staff of 5, including 2 nannies, bookwork and payroll. We would split the responsibilities accordingly. We enjoyed cooking and entertaining.

In addition, Dennis worked hands on and oversaw anything external, blowing walks, painting, structural issues, anything to do with maintenance or construction. During the off-season, we worked on the internal and external maintenance of the estate. This was very expansive.

We wanted the estate to always be prepared and in a state of readiness for the family or guests. We were prepared for their arrival at a moments notice. In addition we wanted the family to enjoy their home and enjoy its splendor. We treated them and their guests, with the considerations to details such as fresh flowers, and warm towels, baskets with fresh cheese and amenities always at the ready.

I worked hands on, and oversaw anything internal as far as staff, housekeeping, laundry, cooking, shopping, errands, and arrangements for children's schedule. I would put together a summer calendar, with daily and hourly commitments for everyone in the family. We were in our element. It was wonderful! And we just adored the family, falling totally in love with them.

We were very aware of boundaries, and did our best to keep things on a very professional level as well. We understood that this was extremely important. When the family was in residence, we were on call 24-7. We worked long hours and were happy to be there for them. We loved our job!

There was a high level of mutual respect and consideration. This is the key to a partnership such as this...this is why we were willing to always go the extra mile for them, regardless of what was expected of us. They were also very generous and kind. But, I think a lot of families in this position do not realize that treating their staff with dignity and respect is the key element in a successful relationship. We also, treated our staff that we oversaw with dignity and respect and encouraged them to be the best. So, it is all encompassing, and again an example of what goes around comes around. We get back what we give, whether we are the giver or receiver. God and the universe bless us according to our intentions and efforts.

In November of 2003, we were fortunate to travel to Europe for this family to train the staff overseas. I am standing in line at the airport, with excitement building, getting ready for an 8-hour flight. I am amazed that I have come this far.

We settle into our seats on the plane and I think of how interesting life can be if we do not give up, and have a trusting and open heart. Thinking of how many years I spent succumbing to panic and fear. What a waste, of my best years. Sighing I am happy that it is far behind me.

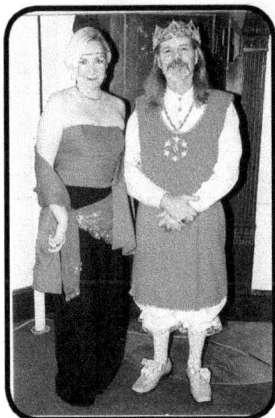

Cast Party with my
brother Ed.

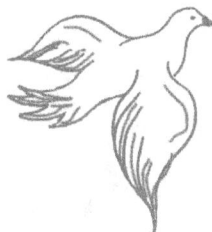

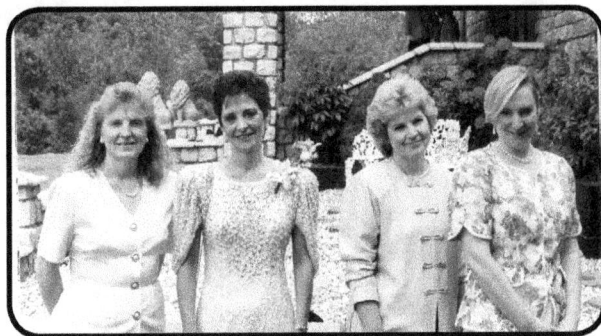

The Reed Sisters,
Kathy, Denise, Carol, and Sharon

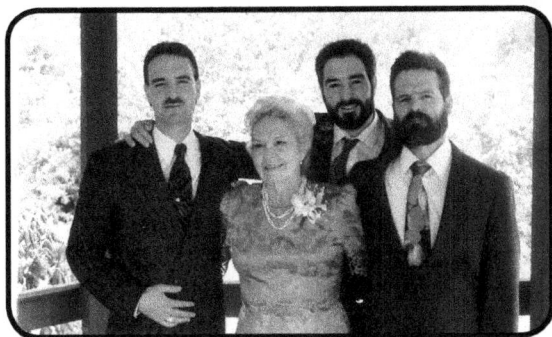

The Reed Brothers
with our Mother.
Mark, Mom, Dan, and Ed.

Men are not prisoners of fate, but only prisoners of their own minds.

Franklin D. Roosevelt

Put To The Test

After we had been in flight for several hours, I look down and comment on what appears to be a blanket of snow over Iceland. Those are clouds my husband tells me with amusement. I am awe struck at the beauty, and the significance of the moment hits me. Never in my wildest dreams did I ever think that I would be capable of living this life or to see the world from this perspective.

I am overwhelmed with the gift of opportunity that was presented to me through our association with this family. I am experiencing things in my life, which would never have been otherwise. I am grateful and humbled to be a part of this.

Our flight lands and, we see a man holding a placard with our names on it. He leads us to a lounge for foreigners where we wait while our luggage is going through customs. After sometime, we are led to a waiting car with a driver and our translator. We are told that they will be at our assistance throughout our stay.

We drive to our employer's main house; we meet and greet the staff and others that we will be working with. We set up a schedule of our intended work related situations and get down to business. The purpose of this trip is to organize their two residences and to train the staff to run their homes in Europe as we do in the States. We are very happy to oblige and accommodate any requests.

We have a very affable and cooperative interpreter, he is very helpful in relating to the staff our different instructions, and we use a lot of sign language. We like the other help, and we get along well, they are considerate and hard working. They also care very much for our employer and want to please him. We set about reorganizing and retraining the households. After three weeks, it is successful. Our employers seem pleased and we are pleased.

Our employer is kind enough to arrange for us to fly out to St. Petersburg for an evening of dinner and Russian Ballet. The next day we see the culturally magnificent, Hermitage, Catherine the Greats' Palace, art museums and Red Square. We are inundated with education, and culture and history. We are shopping on the brick streets with vendors who are hocking their wares.

We are seeing first hand the panhandling that goes on in the streets by very young children. We see the high-end shops that remind me so much of Montreal Canada. The men are handsome, and the women are beautiful and very fashionable. Russia seems to be very modern, not at all what I imagined. To my surprise, it has become very westernized. This was not the Russia that I was expecting.

It is total culture shock. We see the expanse of years of history right in front of us. There are the older women with babushkas walking the streets and shopping and then the totally modern and stylistic younger generation walking right beside them, it was fascinating. I was thrilled at the experience of it all! It is definitely a different Russia today than even 20 years ago. I was surprised at how advanced they were in some ways in technology, and how a lot of the people were multi-lingual, this too was unexpected. One afternoon, we were standing in line at a café, and I looked at the young man that was waiting on me. A bit perplexed as to how to order, I pointed to the food items that I had been eyeing, and said reluctantly " I no speak Russian" He looked at me, very blasé, and answered very clearly "So speak English!"

We are wrapping up our work for the day, getting ready for our weekend trip to St. Petersburg, and the news is ablaze with the Chechnyan take over in a St. Petersburg Theater, OH NO! Terrorists have taken people hostage in a theater and the demands must be met or people will die. What a world we live in. is it safe anywhere? With 9/11 in 2001 and now this thoughts of panic and anxiety begin to creep in. The world is not a safe place to be. This is right in the heart of where we will be traveling to the next day. I begin to feel a familiar foreboding, and that terror of not being safe.

Watching the telecasts, we determine to continue with our plans, regardless of this latest news. I refuse to let this latest development stifle my progress. I get a grip on my anxiety and do not panic, remembering not to feed fear-into-fear. I have a slight sense of what if? but trusting in my higher power and the plans, and the designs of the universe, I decide to move forward with so what and remembering again, not to feed fear-into-fear. I refuse to let this feeling of panic control me. This was too great an opportunity to pass up, a once in a lifetime. We went to the Ballet and enjoyed it immensely. It was a fabulous and a memorable evening.

On our flight back to the States, looking out the window, thinking this was definitely one of the highlights of my life. This experience was exhilarating! I am acutely aware of what would have been missed, if I had allowed panic and fear to still be a part of my life. So, blessed am I. I stay diligent and determined enough in the past to work at overcoming this "terror".

It is a turning point, being out of the throws of this debilitating and life-altering affliction. And to have had the experience to associate with, and work for considerate and appreciative people at this point in life, forever grateful!

We continued to work with this family for five years. We were with them through major milestones in their lives. Births, deaths, christenings, large and festive holidays, Christmas, New Years, Easter, Thanksgiving. Family vacations and travel, and church functions steeped deep in tradition. Later our service included building renovations, hiring chefs, and acquiring large yachts.

We had a professional and cordial relationship with the secretaries, and his assistant in Europe. We were in touch on a monthly basis with our book work and financial statements and estate issues as well as family requests.

We shared in their sorrows through the loss of loved ones. We prepared and arranged for their generous entertaining of friends and relatives and social functions. It was heartwarming to watch them interact with each other as a family. It was a joy to watch the children grow up and their family expand. They traveled all over the country and the world. It was fast paced and a whirlwind of wonderful experiences.

It was not without its challenges from time to time, but this is to be expected when you work so closely and intimately with others. All in all, it was a mutually satisfying relationship. We have very fond memories, the highest regard, and a lifetime of gratitude. I developed a close relationship with the family senior matriarch. She was very spiritual and wise, she was a dear, and will always hold a special place in my heart.

In the summer of 2004, our employer and his wife graciously offer us a weekend on their yacht for Dennis Birthday. They encourage us to invite friends or relatives and to enjoy! On a beautiful July evening, with a clear and star-studded sky, we cruise the New York harbor with friends, the captain and crew, and then we dock for dinner. What a lovely gesture! Life was good.

I attribute this experience of being on the outside looking in, in part to my ability to be able to build trust once again in family relationships, even with all the dynamics that come into play. To understand that with all of our different personalities, we can still learn from one another and respect, and accept our differences. It was a gift. We continued to work in this capacity for another year.

When the family was not in residence and we were not on call Dennis and I got involved in ballroom dancing, I took of all things belly dancing for exercise and Dennis took art classes, to brush up on his already accomplished technique.

We had a social network of friends that we became close with. We had yearly vacations and a generous amount of time off. We were invited to gatherings and our life was full. We had dinner parties in our own separate apartment, which our employer encouraged. In turn we took very meticulous care of the estate. We were acutely aware of the importance of representing the family with respect and dignity.

In the fall of 2005, after an extremely busy and long season with the family, we get a call from Dennis sister, his mother is dying, and they do not know how much time she has. We arranged to travel to Massachusetts. After much planning and determining our future, we decide that maybe we should think about being closer to our families.

Upon returning to New York, after Dennis mother's funeral, we find that the family that we work for is considering spending more time in Europe, and spending less time in the States. We are not certain of our place in all of this. Perhaps it is time to move on. Circumstances are changing in all of our lives. It has been an awesome experience. We worked hard and learned a lot and now life is moving forward. We are getting older, and time does not stand still. Perhaps it is time to look at our own priorities.

After long discussions with our employer, we all come to the sad agreement to part ways. We spend two months getting things in order for them for a smooth transition. We care deeply about them, and want to leave on the best terms. We pack up five years of possessions acquired, and wonderful memories. With mixed feelings of sadness, reluctance, and hugs, we say our good byes. We sincerely wish each other well for future endeavors.

On a cool brisk November morning, we drive a truck with our New York life neatly packed in boxes, and drive pensively towards Vermont. We have spent five years of our lives with this family as a priority. This was a new feeling, to be free of this type of commitment. I have mixed feelings about this. Although, I am happy to be reuniting with my own sons in Vermont, whom I have missed immensely.

The first week that we are back in Vermont, I look out the window and see a fine layer of snowflakes starting to blanket the ground. It feels so wonderful to be back North, although we had no idea what our future would hold. We spend time with our sons, and revel in the close proximity to family.

In 2006, we welcomed in the New Year with gaiety and hopes for a productive and prosperous future. We had planned to be working in real estate with my sister Kathy and her husband. After a successful beginning, this proved to be non productive as the market was beginning to lag. After six months of starts and stops, we decide to send our resumes out once again. Well, we are older. It is not as easy to secure a job once you hit fifty.

It was a very daunting and disappointing process. What an awakening, there does not seem to be the interest in our skills as previously. How could that be?

It is amazing how quickly we forget where we have been. It's almost as if life has to shake us up a little bit, and knock us off our pedestals to remind us where we have come from. Maybe we need a good set back to remember the lessons we have learned and to learn new ones.

In 2007 the inability to secure any promising career opportunities in Vermont or elsewhere, brings us back to Springfield, Mass where my husband and I grew up. We are now immersed with family and friends from years ago. This brings new challenges of negotiating all the slippery slope of the past. Well, sometimes we manage, and sometimes we don't.

We go right back to what we knew best, property management. Acquiring buildings that need rehab and renovating, and we start to build income property and a tenant base. We are in business yet again. We invite my brother Danny who owns a tile company to become a business partner in the real estate and together he and my husband keep each other employed. I believe that he has attained his own recovery, I am proud of him.

It is dejà vu again. It is reminiscent of the early 1990s. We are in real estate and the market is crashing. The country is heading for a recession. I have to figure out a way to contribute that is substantial. We have invested a lot of our savings into trying to help our children get on their feet at this point in their lives. Our oldest son Justin is the technical director of a theater in New Bedford, Mass, and engaged to be married. Todd, our middle son, is working in the food service industry; he and his wife Sarah have just blessed us with our first grandchild. Our youngest son Evan is working successfully in real estate management but, wondering how long his job is secure. It seems that the financial struggles are never ending!

We have gone from making six figures a year, and being very comfortable and secure, to wondering if we could weather this latest crisis. I decide to go back to the familiar, health care and renew my license as a LNA through the Red Cross. I take the spring semester classes with the hopes of securing a clinical position. Pleased with becoming re-certified, I continue to work in private care through an agency. I am encouraged with the possibility of professional opportunities and doing well.

In 2008, I apply for a position at a major hospital, and am very interested in working clinically. Not hearing from anyone for sometime, I begin to think that it is my age, who wants to hire someone for 12 hour shifts who is fifty something? Although, I have lots of energy, excellent references, and proven ability in health care, it continues to be a long process. I call every week for three months to check on the status of hiring positions.

In the spring of 2008, I receive a call from my brother Eddy, he tells me that the community theater group that he works with is holding auditions for the upcoming theater production of the movie Holes. Would I be interested? Well, yes, I say tentatively. I had always dreamed of the opportunity to try my hand at theater, but lacked the confidence to even give it a try. It's now or never! I decide to go for it. It will be a good diversion, while waiting to hear of job possibilities.

I arrange to audition for a part. The day of the audition I arrive with my CD in tow. We were told to come prepared to sing. I knew just what I was going to sing! I had my favorite song by Martina McBride Broken Wing I had this down pat. I knew it by heart! This was the story of my life.

I walk into the rehearsal room of an old building. I sign in and begin to watch the others auditioning, uh oh, they seem a lot more experienced. I do not think this is going to fly. I will never be able to do this, but, to my amazement, I belt out the song, and actually sound good! How about that?

I was a bit nervous, but not overwhelmed. I was offered the part as Stanley's Mother, and with my confidence growing, commit to the summer show.

All goes well, and we start rehearsal. I am definitely a fish out of water with these theater veterans. But, struggle through a new experience in breaking a barrier to fear. All the while, remembering my mantras "Just go with it, jump in, just do it, do not feed fear-into-fear, who cares? So what, it's ok to fail" etc etc no one is perfect, it does not matter. Have fun!

The show opened on a warm summer evening in June to a full house. I am standing back stage waiting for our cue, my stomach is in knots. I am VERY nervous. I have a monologue to recite and am terrified that I will forget the words mid sentence. In my mind, I keep saying "I can do this, I can do this." I am very familiar with this feeling of fear. I can move through this, but this is a different type of fear. There is an excitement as well as fear.

The curtain rises, the lights go up, and I am on stage. I do not see the audience. I perform as if I have been here before. During the performance, I am much calmer than anticipated. I finish with my performance, and walk off stage. I am ecstatic coming through another hurdle of fear. While I am mingling afterwards with the other cast members. I am the only one who knows what a monumental success this truly was for me. Elated and very proud of this moment, you go girl!

In July of 2008, I pick up the phone to make one last call to H.R. After a few rings I hear someone answer. I tell her that I am following up on my resume, and did she have any information regarding positions.

Well, I just happen to be working on TA positions as we speak, she says. There is an opening on the respiratory floor, is this something you would be interested in? Absolutely! I say, happy to have finally gotten a positive response. I will set up an appointment with the nurse manager for 1:00 p.m. on Tues she says. Emphatically I commit to being there and hang up the phone.

Enthusiastically I arrive for my interview with an air of professionalism. Walking down the hall, I am struck by all the complex equipment. All procedures that TAs are responsible for are entered into computers immediately. There is an array of oxygen and trachea equipment that is perplexing to me. This is unfamiliar territory.

I enter the nurse mangers office and introduce myself. We shake hands, and she proceeds to look over my resume, educational background, and references. She has a list of hypothetical questions that she asks me. What would I do in such and such a situation? After the initial interview, she gives me a tour of the unit, and introduces me to other staff. She thanks me for my time, and says she will make a decision in a few days.

I wait with anticipation to hear from the hospital. The call finally comes, and they offer a position at a starting salary I am pleased with. After all, not being experienced on a clinical respiratory floor, but the nurse manager assures me this is not a problem, they will train me and provide opportunities for education and will have a 2-3 month orientation period to become familiar with the complexities of the floor. Terrific. I am thrilled.

I begin orientation with high hopes. The hospital promotes what appears to be genuine interest in their employees and their success. They place a high regard on encouraging the new employees to be the best that they can be. They promote hands on learning and teamwork. I feel confident my orientation and education by my preceptor (teacher) and other staff will be a fair and respectful environment. They have zero tolerance for employee harassment. This is a good thing. They really promote mutual respect among employees, wonderful!

Management assures me that the other employees that are training new employees have their best interest at heart. I am confident at the end of my orientation, I will have a solid foundation to do my job and do it well. I relax and trust in this process.

On the first day of clinical, I am placed in the respiratory unit. There is so much information to take in. I express to my preceptor, I would like to become familiar with the computer programs and the different oxygen delivery systems, which this is all new to me and she says, in time.

The new technology for respirators, and patients with tracheae is amazing. I have a ton of questions, about a ton of things. I get the impression that this may not be a good thing. Even though, we are told that we should ask questions. I sense impatience, with my curiosity. So, I try to suppress my questions.

There are at least twenty Doctors, nurses, and TAs on any given day, on our unit. We have a nurse manager, a nurse educator, and a charge nurse, RNs for each side of each unit with 4 Patients each. And TAs who have 8-9 patients each, sometimes more, Phew! That's interesting, the TAs have the most patients to care for. Well, I am sure they all work together in a team effort.

The five weeks of my orientation on the medical side are successful with one preceptor. My orientation is to be completed by a transfer to the respiratory side. I begin to sense inconsistency pertaining to my training. I am now working with several different preceptors. They have a lot of different personalities, and understanding of skills and protocol. There are many different dynamics. Another hoop to jump through in the realm of dysfunction. Another maze, to navigate my way through and another life lab. Here we go again, Oh no!

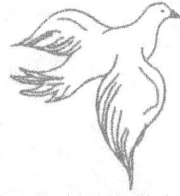

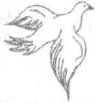

Endurance is not just the ability to bear a hard thing, but to turn it into glory.

William Barclay

Endurance

It became very apparent to me that regardless of how well I did my job or worked hard, or how respectful, diplomatic, and dignified I approached my coworkers this was going to be another lesson in endurance. What a lesson it became. This was a tight group and I was the outsider. No problem! This was familiar ground! I was very aware of the dysfunction all around me. People are not even aware of, but in reality dysfunction is often masked in judgmental behaviors that are counterproductive to well being.

Prejudice • Competitiveness • Sarcasm • Rudeness Jealousy • Self-righteousness • Taunting • Insensitivity • Insincerity • Judgment• Superior •Unkindness • Dishonesty Impatience • Criticism •Lack of perception • Misrepresentation •Verbal abuse • Perfection •Inconsistency • Misinterpretation • Emotional abuse • Pride • Lack of compassion • Lack of forgiveness • lack of acceptance

This is also predominate, (bullying), in schools, even as adults. How can we expect our children to learn healthy ways of interacting if we keep repeating our own dysfunctions and prejudices in the workplace as adults? It is all around us, we see the struggling with this in every field. Behavior that is not centered in an open, honest, and sincere heart is what creates all of our social and emotional problems. It is the core of dysfunction and failures.

It seems like lifetimes ago that I first became aware of family dysfunction and the result of panic and anxiety. The truth is we are always going to be surrounded in this big beautiful world of ours by different personalities. Sometimes we click and other times we do not. Through it all, I have come to understand that we are definitely each other's teachers, and if we are centered we become each other's keepers. Our world and society need spiritual healing.

Sometimes we are successful in our endeavors and other times we are not. Sometimes life lessons are a big part of the way things transpire. And sometimes we are fortunate enough to experience others through satisfying and centered experiences.

We do not always have to win nor do we need to always be right. There are times when we will never know the reasons for the actions. Sometimes, regardless of how well we do something or how perfect it appears to be, it is just not meant to be. There is not always a silver-lining, perhaps the universe has a message, if we are attuned to seeing the lesson.

On a grey rainy day, the weather reflective of my mood. I am sitting on the shuttle headed for my morning shift at the hospital. With a sense of gloom, wondering if I will be able to keep a positive attitude. Having worked very hard, I did not anticipate such a struggle. It is not the work, because this was truly enjoyable. I begin to realize how difficult this is becoming for me. I do not feel supported and feel there is a lot of my training that is being missed. My preceptors are not forthcoming with information. I try to stay positive and professional. I begin to feel the undercurrent of that personality thing. Oh boy, here we go again!

Preparing for my morning shift and I am told that I will be working with a new preceptor to complete my training on the respiratory side. She will instruct me for the remaining four days of my orientation. This is not a normal policy to work with several different employees in a two week period of time. On orientation one generally works with one preceptor, two at the most, to prevent any confusion in what has been instructed, and to also allow for a supportive and fair learning environment.

This was not my experience. She does not instruct me, but only evaluates me. Where is the consistency that was promised? This is very confusing, they do not seem to know what the other has instructed or evaluated. My training seems so disorganized. But, of course my managers will straighten this out. I am sure of it. On this particular morning upon completing my vitals, Miss hoity toity (my new Preceptor) comes sauntering down the hall with a slight smirk on her face. You are going to drown you just do not get it! She says with a sneer and sarcasm in her heavy accent. Oh my, another Godzilla, lucky me.

She proceeds to tell me I should have all of my vitals on patients completed and entered into the computer by 7:30 in the morning. I had them done by 8:00 Now, this is a respiratory unit with patients who are on ventilators and tracheas, and I am doing complete mouth care on 8 patients as well as vitals, and several of them are in isolation. How is that possible? Especially when you do not start until 7:15? I would think that patient care not time management would be a priority. And, wait a minute, I am still learning all the equipment, I reason, this does not sound right. I try to be gracious with her instructions and, I say nothing about my thoughts, but agree that I will work on time management.

My preceptor (trainer) is an experienced employee, however (not a supervisor). She continues with what I consider unreasonable and inconsistent evaluations, they do not seem to make sense. Not to worry, my managers will see through this and intercede on my behalf. I am confident that at our next meeting, all this will be addressed and the discrepancies surrounding my training will be cleared up. After all, I am the one who is training, far be it for me to question my preceptors approach, until I have all the facts, right?

I do my best to brave the unhealthy attitudes that are all around me. I am comfortable enough in my own skin and determined to succeed. I put my best foot forward, and I continue to try to learn with acceptance. I have the uncanny feeling that I have been here before, many times in my life. What is the purpose? I mean it is everywhere, this incredible dysfunctional way of people interacting.

So much for my illusion of support, it was not to be. But, at this point, I understand that this is life and ride it out. How resilient I have become. My understanding of detachment and hard work at overcoming my dysfunction allows me to know that I will be able to over come this and detach from this onslaught. It felt like I was in a den of wolves.

When people in the world start their stuff it spreads like wild fire, specially when in large groups. And if you are the focus, your toast! Anyone can put a positive or negative spin on any situation. So, if the majority rules in dysfunction, forget about it! You know the glass half empty or half full analogy. It's all the same, but one is viewed from a positive viewpoint and the other a negative viewpoint. It is all relative to how we look at things.

Unfortunately for me, or fortunately, depending on how you look at it, my last two days of orientation, I had an unplanned event. I was sick and there was no way that I could work in patient care. So, that was it for me! I was dismissed, no explanation, warning or meeting to determine an alternate plan for the rest of orientation. Nothing that was it! But, once again, my body was responding to my thoughts.

I am rarely sick at this point in my life, however I became sick and run down. My sight was affected, no doubt, because I did not want to see the reality and the truth of what was going on around me! I know better this time being seasoned enough to pay attention to what my body is telling me. Spiritually there is a lesson for me. What the lesson is, is a mystery to me. I am supposed to be seeing- through this latest challenge of mine. We continually receive unconsciously the unspoken messages that are being sent out in our direction by others. If that interaction is not uplifting or emotionally healthy, it wears our spirit down and eventually it shows itself physically.

Our hearts become heavy and it saps our energy. If our experiences are not mutually satisfying, emotionally, spiritually, and physically, we are wasting our time and it creates a void in our life. Hopefully, we get the lesson that we are supposed to be learning and quickly! So, that we can move on and get on with life and presumably more lessons, gracefully.

However, at the time I was discharged the hospital was laying off a large number of employees that same week and there were budget cuts etc. I was told that many of the unit managers were being told they were over budget and needed to find ways to resolve that. Isn't that interesting? This made me question the validity of my dismissal. And I proceeded to fire off letters, to managers and supervisors, and human resources, all in the name of fairness you see. Although, I am sure they do not agree. Because, if management is aware of some the practices of their supervisors, perhaps it will help future potential employees to be successful, I assume with an indignant air to my convictions.

I send off my letters and I express my viewpoint. I state that I believe their evaluation system by other peers is open to abuse and perhaps they should be aware of this. It is a shame that they spend the amount of time, money, and resources on potentially good employees that are undermined before they even get off the ground because of the misguided critique of another employee. And on and on, I continue to make my point in writing. But, who cares! I finally accept there is a lesson here.

Shortly after my dismissal, I am on the phone with L. I ask her if we can meet for a session in biorhythm. I proceed to question the validity of my dismissal. I am incensed about the dismissal under such circumstances. This does not reflect my overall positive performance I tell her. This is so unjust!

Perhaps, it was not the right floor for me-but this should have been honestly discussed. Perhaps it was personalities, or budget cuts, or because I was inquisitive. I certainly did not deserve to be dismissed in such a way. I tell her I am going to contact everyone in a supervisory position so that they will become aware of some of the management practices that are undermining potentially good employees, before they even get off the ground.

I would have been very competent if I had been supported in my orientation. This evaluation system that they have on some floors is open to abuse. It is only as good as the person doing the evaluating. Laughing, isn't this the purpose of our life's journey? All the lessons are through the people with whom we interact. What do you think the lesson is? I say to L.

Never in a million years would it have occurred to me a

person would be let go in such a manner. I have excellent references in health care and I generally have good work attendance and get along well with coworkers. Do you think it has something to do with all the layoffs and the budget cuts? I ask. Maybe it was my signature red lipstick I say interjecting some humor. Unfortunately some women are threatened by others who take pride in their appearance, oh well, wouldn't be the first time! For heaven sakes, it's always something. I know, she says, "Life sure is crazy!"

It is at this exact moment that I have a fleeting inspiration. Maybe it is" time "for me to tell my story. This is the purpose, because if I had never been so ungraciously let go, I would not have been humbled enough and motivated enough to put my story in writing. I have overcome agoraphobia, anxiety, and fear, going on to do amazing and incredible things. Experiences I would not have thought possible. I have stood the endurance of difficult challenges and have survived and excelled. So if my experience in some way is an inspiration to others then I am listening to the messages of God and the universe and I will pass it on.

The lesson is to accept the things that happen to us in our life as a gift. It may not always have a silver lining, but it is not always a detriment either. Behind every heartache and struggle perhaps is a blessing, just waiting for the right moment to reveal itself. In my case, the blessing was the opportunity to share my story.

If I had not had the hospital experience. I would not have questioned the purpose, and I would not have been motivated to put my struggle with panic and anxiety on paper, in the hopes of helping others. I assumed it was behind me and that is where it would stay. I never looked back.

I decide to visit my son Todd, his wife, and my new grandson in Vermont. Our relationship has been a bit strained. I suppose because of his perception of his upbringing. I long ago went passed all the stuff regarding my relationships, but I suspect that he is still working on his. I learned a long time ago that we all need to work through our past in our own way.

I hope that he is open to listening to me because I have something to share. Calling him on the phone and telling him of my dismissal, I apologize to him for being so judgmental when he lost his job a few years before.

I distinctly remember telling him and his brothers when they were younger in a work situation you do not gossip, do your job and your best to get along with others. Try to be cooperative, and helpful with coworkers, be on time, and remember to smile! Then there is no reason to be fired! People will have no reason to dislike you or undermine you. I was wrong, forgetting the dynamics of personalities that sometimes come into play.

We spend a few days visiting. I delight in the smiles and the giggles of this new little guy, my grandson. He is handsome and strong and a blessing. It brings me back to when my children were young. Thinking of those precious moments, I sometimes missed with my own babies during my struggling. How far ahead of the game that they are as parents and how lucky they are. There is happiness to be with my son in an effort to put the past behind us and move forward. He is a very good father. I am proud of all three of my boys. Somehow, we all made it through or did we?

After returning from Vermont I am on the phone with "L" telling her of my latest inspiration and I think seriously of putting together a manuscript. Telling her how I thought one of the other reasons for losing my job was to learn a few more lessons in humility, among other things. But, it also was an opportunity for me to reach out to others and to share recovery in a way. Life never ceases to amaze me.

So, what will you do now? She asks. I am going to use this time to reflect, visit my children and grandchild in Vermont for Christmas, and then fly out to visit my mother and sister Carol in Florida, in February. Maybe I will pursue my certification in addiction counseling. That's wonderful! There is life beyond the medical profession after all, she says a bit wryly, who knew. Exactly, I say to her, who knew?

The important thing is that I did not fold. Shuffled my cards and played the game. Only I was aware of the true significance of my accomplishments in that statement. How grateful to have overcome and to have persevered through some very difficult and seemingly impossible struggles.

Although, there will be more lessons, I feel truly blessed! Because today, I do not have to be perfect and there is nothing to fear. Through these challenges, I am learning and growing.

In February of 2009, I invited my son his wife and grandchild to move in with us for a short time. It did not work lasting four months. Once again I came face to face with the consequences of addiction. I let the tears flow and then I let go. I knew what was needed.

I scheduled some therapy sessions to work this heartache through. It is important to deal with emotions and sadness in the now. It is important to talk it through from a different perspective and come to terms with painful experiences in a healthy way. I attend a few 12 step meetings to reconnect with the lessons I have learned and a new resolve to consciously maintain recovery in all areas. I make a mental note to start taking better care of my self on all levels, because it seems I have lost my focus through these latest disappointments. I am very aware of the need to stay spiritually centered and pay attention to my health physically. Why did I start smoking again? I make a vow to give it up completely! I know better than to give into life's stresses this way.

A few weeks later, my sister Denise, and I discuss our family and how differently our upbringing was perceived. Why are you bringing all these things up now? She asks. I explain I was just referring to how we carry emotional pain from our life's experiences in our bodies until we let it surface in a constructive way so that we can heal. We all need to be aware as to how we were affected in our childhoods in order to be healthy adults.

Who can explain memory? And how one person can be so traumatized by some experiences and others seem to breeze right through life, without so much as a backward glance, nothing seems to faze them.

"Well you may have grown up in an alcoholic home, but I did not!" She responds. "I was out of the house by the time Dads drinking progressed. I did not experience what you did."

Ok I say, knowing that we all have our own history to deal with, she has hers, and I have mine. I am reminded of how deep denial can be. I am more concerned at this point for my own children and how their (our) history has impacted them.

I understand that I am powerless over others and how they conduct their lives, see the world or see me. I cannot "fix" someone else. I cannot make them happy only they can find their own happiness. I know my intentions towards my son and his family and others came from the purest part of myself and what pained me the most is it was not received this way.

I accept the fact again, that we all need to learn our own lessons. There have been times in my life when giving to my loved ones in any form was not seen as a gift. Hopefully someday, they will see these efforts with the love and joy it was intended to bring. Sometimes what we think is helping others only becomes a source of resentment depending on their mindset. Sometimes we have to step aside and let others learn their lessons in their own way and their own time. As hard as it is sometimes we all need this choice and dignity.

We all make mistakes. How do we work these things out if anger is the dominant emotion? Nothing ever gets resolved. I needed to remove myself from an environment of anger and lack of forgiveness. Our thinking is clouded by the past and the present cannot enter. It is how we think!

Resolution in relationships happens with clear thinking, free of drug and alcohol addictions. Otherwise, our thoughts and memories are muddled, clouded and distorted.

We need to adjust our thinking and get unstuck from the experiences of the past they are over. And open our self up to new ways of interacting and dealing with others. We can only do that for our self, we cannot do it for someone else.

If a relationship needs healing, we can only do our part and need to be met half way. It does not mean staying in a relationship that is abusive or unhealthy.

I have forgiven people in my life and the past, My fear is the past has not forgiven me, it is my hope that these things that keep repeating in my life will become apparent as to the reason. Could this be another lesson in endurance? Humility? Patience? Forgiveness? Ahhhh...acceptance! Let go and let God.

It's also possible that at some point, the past will no longer matter, and love and forgiveness (will) override all the hurts. Sometimes regardless of what we do some relationships do not work. I allowed myself to feel the sadness and loss for now.

The traumas of our history, our childhood, our parenting, life in general can rise to the surface of our lives when we least expect it transference is a mystifying occurrence. It's as if the disjointed memories of the past become a reality in the present. If one becomes stuck in the past, memories are often misconstrued with misinformation that takes on a life of its own. And every time this memory is brought up to recall there is a re-traumatizing. It is as if it really happened, just the way your mind remembers (true or not), with the intensity that is felt. False memory becomes a reality.

It's self-abuse to keep recalling our history, without constructive steps through therapy, to put things in perspective, forgive, and move on in life.

It often fuels misplaced anger, and we become very sick emotionally and physically. There are often things that are missing from our recall, things that would explain behavior. Things that would help us to see differently and to be able to let go, surrender.

I tell you there is nothing in the world,
Only an ocean of tomorrows, a sky of tomorrows.

~from "Prairie" by Carl Sandburg

This is where recovery and talk therapy is so important, to be released from our own memories and put them in perspective, otherwise, they will haunt us and permeate every area of our lives. We benefit so much from releasing the hurts of the past as we remember them. Once we put the memories, in perspective they have no emotional charge and they have no power over us. Then we are free and emotionally clear to move on in life. When one is unable or unwilling to make peace with and forgive the hurts and grievances of a life gone by it is almost impossible to rise above it and live in the now.

Endurance

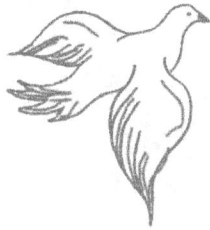

"Your children come through you. They are not you."

~Kahlil Gibrahn

The Grief of Addiction:

A mother's perspective

We often face this dilemma with our adult children, who were exposed to all the dysfunction and dynamics of addiction before our own recovery. When they become adults, the cycle begins to repeat, if we have not been fortunate to break the cycle before it does the most damage to our families.

With the gift of recovery, I had intentions of imparting love, kindness, compassion, and tolerance into my relationships. Imagine my surprise as we interacted and I began to be drawn into the drama and dysfunction of the past. How can this be? Where is the recovery I possessed? It was through much sorrow and grief I realized we cannot give recovery to anyone else; we can only sustain our own balance.

We will very quickly be drawn into the craziness again when we are exposed to direct blame, guilt, anger, and hostility from others. We need to forgive one another and move on in our lives with humility and gratitude otherwise, we are traveling against the wind. We are not moving in the direction that God and the universe designed for us.

For a mother this is particularly heart wrenching, when addiction and dysfunction have such a hold on your adult children, that you are the focus of their anger and rage about the past. You are their focus if they have not worked through their own history, even though you have. It is without a doubt the most heartbreaking experience a mother can face. Regardless of how much love and energy that we give to our children, we sometimes lose them either emotionally or physically to the disease. This loss can be for a season or sometimes completely, it is after all their choice. I love all of my children deeply and it is my hope and prayer that they will heal and work it through. I believe that they will.

They need to walk their own path and work out their own lives as they deem appropriate. We may want to save them from the clutches of this spiral, but, they have their own walk to walk. It is a process as all of our lessons and struggles are.

"Sadness is a wall between two gardens." Kahil Gibran

Hopefully as I move on in life and my adult children move on in theirs. I pray that they will be able to break the chains of addiction and dysfunction and see their way clear; so it will not impact another generation of innocence.

This I believe is our destiny, to bring together our families and relationships. We need to be willing to let go and forgive the past. It is my belief that my part is opening the door to reconciliation and healing in my relationships. This is the best that I can do. I need to be with others who are healthy and striving to be centered, be balanced in my efforts, so that I stay on the path of emotional wellness and recovery.

These last few years have been full of surprises, heartaches, and twists and turns. It seems as though life is moving at lightning speed. The lessons and challenges are coming faster than I can imagine in rapid succession.

I decide to further my education in understanding addiction and attend Westfield State University. I graduated with a certification in alcohol and drug counseling and did an internship at a rehabilitation center for the addicted and homeless. I am humbled and resolved that this is truly a very cunning affliction. Some make it and rise above while there are others who battle for a life time. I believe there is hope and I will continue to share and to listen. I do not have all the answers. But, I understand the struggle for wellbeing.

Millions are suffering from anxiety and agoraphobia. Medications are prescribed more often than not, recovery is possible without long term medications. I know because I fought this battle and won.

Somewhere in the cosmos, at some point in time we were appointed to our life's lessons. I truly believe, we are each other's teachers, and for some reason as they say the heart has its reasons that mind doesn't know. And so we were designed to take this journey together for a higher purpose. Our purpose is to try to understand God, one another and our place in this universe. And so it goes.

Harvest Time

Country women's faces wear, a clean, apron majesty
Beside, which city faces seem a glossy travesty.

Country faces bear, the marks of life's deep rhythm with a minimum of fuss and no self pity, for this cause I left the city.

When my time comes of finalness, Id like others to see in me...not how much youth I have retained, but how I have let go, to gather what I know.....How much living I have gained.

I want my face to look like theirs, with eyes alight with bravery and lines like prayers.

Michael Drury

Summary

Cause and Effect; We are impacted by our environment and the people that we interact with on a daily basis.

We are what our past has been, never underestimate the power of our experiences, emotionally, physically, verbally.

Counseling and treatment is essential in coming to terms with the hurts and traumas of the past, by talking it through.

Spiritually we need to connect with God as our source. It is our purpose in life.

Letting go, forgiveness is the best gift that we can give to our self and others, it sets us free. Making amends to others.

Dealing with anxiety whatever you are feeling do not fight it. Do not feed fear-into-fear. Turn what ifs, into so what!

Fear it is the fear of the fear that is so terrifying.

Desensitizing through proactive therapy is imperative in ones recovery. Slowly, facing the fear and the underlying conflict.

Depression is often caused by wrong thinking! I believe that this is the cause of chemical imbalance...which then causes panic, anxiety and despondency. It also, can have an underlying physiological component for many different reasons, but this too can be turned around. We need to get to the source. Diet, medications, allergies....over indulgence in alcohol or drugs.

Stress changes our metabolism and emotions. The way we think causes the stress chemical imbalance, not the other way around! We can change our physiological responses by how we think!

Breaking free from Panic Anxiety
and
Agoraphobia

Excerpts from my journal after my stay at Spofford Hall Sept 1983

Alcoholism as I understood through 12 Steps

A. Alcoholism is a three fold disease, mental, physical , and spiritual. Our parents were victims of the disease, which ends in insanity and or death. Learning about and understanding the disease is the beginning of *the gift of forgiveness*.

B. We learn the three Cs---we didn't cause it, we cant control it, and we cant cure it.

C. We learn to put the focus on ourselves and to be good to ourselves.

D. We learn to detach with love, and give ourselves and others tough love.

E. We use the al anon slogans:" Let go and let God" Easy does it " One Day at a time" Keep it Simple" Live and Let Live" Using these slogans helps us begin to lead our day to day lives in a new way.

F. We learn to feel our feelings, to accept them and express them, and to build our self esteem.

G. Through working the steps, we learn to accept the disease, We realize that:

Our lives have become unmanageable and we are powerless over the disease and the alcoholic. As we become willing to admit our defects and our sick thinking, We are able to change our attitudes and to turn our reactions into actions. By working the program daily, admitting we are powerless. We become to believe eventually in the spirituality of the program. That there is a solution other than ourselves, the group, a higher power...God as we understand him. By sharing our experiences, relating to others, welcome new comers, serving our group (s) we build self esteem.

H.   We learn to love ourselves, in this way we are able to love others in a healthy way.

I.   We have telephone therapy with people we relate to-very helpful at all times, not just when problems arise. We need others to talk things through with.

J.   By applying the serenity prayer to our daily lives, we begin to change the sick attitudes we acquired in childhood.

Serenity Prayer

God grant me the serenity to accept the things I cannot change. Courage to change the things I can And the wisdom to know the difference

The treatment center and 12 step meetings were a beginning of my awareness as to the affects of the disease of alcoholism in my life.....and even more importantly it gave me an immense education as to my background, and the generational affects..and how indeed, we are influenced as to who we are and what we are, by our environment. Perhaps the way we perceive it, is not necessarily the way it is.

Journal notes 1980's

Can you Trust Your Emotions?
It is my conviction that agoraphobia is an emotional bondage masking itself in physical symptoms (panic attacks) from
religious, sexual, and spiritual conflicts as well as relationship
issues. Which in effect renders a person hostage to his emotions?

A very real physical occurrence brought on by stress, the
chemical changes that take place in the brain that can cause
panic. Where do these spiritual, religious, and sexual conflicts
come from? Well meaning , but misguided role models, auto
suggestion, from opinions that are not correct or distorted
hearsay, sick people (alcoholic or otherwise) that we loved or
thought we loved in growing up years, or now. Result, strife,
confusion, mixed messages, inner turmoil, and denial, unable
to face reality of the situation; by stifling, suppressing, stuff-
ing real feelings. Unwilling to admit that it's all wrong!

An inner voice is crying to believe differently and our hearts
tell us differently. We are afraid to look at the reality of our life
(denial). Consequently agoraphobia and anxiety attacks result
as the whirlwind of emotions of anger, guilt, frustration, and
resentment at ourselves and others.

It all has to do with the way the way we think, the way we
perceive things and the way we perceive things may not necessarily be the way things truly are but, only the way it appears
to us. This is where re educating our thinking and how we
view the world and our life's circumstances is extremely helpful in balancing our thinking to begin to get well. When we are
not under this stress of emotion, the brain chemistry balances
itself, and our world looks differently to us.

The key is to view the simple truths in life without all the condemnation. Life was not meant to be full of fear. We want to have healthy views and perspectives. We can do that by looking at the simple truths in life that others have come to understand, and by stepping into their experiences we can make our own decisions in our lives. We can take what we want, and leave the rest, experience is the best teacher. Sometimes we benefit from others attitudes about life. It is not so complicated we make it so difficult. We do not need to have so much drama!

Yet I do believe that some people have a genetic predisposition. There is controversy about agoraphobia or any type of imbalance as being a chemical imbalance. It is my conviction that the chemical imbalance does not cause the depression rather the depression (wrong thinking) causes the chemical imbalance.

Most people are living an illusion pertaining to their lives and they may not be aware of it. We all live in our heads!

Depression
Wrong thinking causes depression. It is brought on by distorted opinions and interactions with others over a period-of-time. Which results in mental assassination? Our thinking becomes imbalanced, which brings on depression, and then a chemical released in the brain almost as if it is short circuiting with all the different messages it is receiving at once. Turmoil with our inner thoughts and at times even thinking about long ago, unconsciously, brings on panic attacks.

The attack will subside once the person feels safe, so it is evident to me that we can control our brain chemistry and functions, by how we think and view circumstances. Which takes training, reeducation and therapy.

Wrong thinking causes chemical imbalance. Our brains are

like computers and memory and thought are a very complex. It can replay repeatedly long ago happenings and become a train wreck. When we are in emotional turmoil or conflict our brain short circuits. If our body is in a weakened state, run down, under stress, or at high intense stress levels, or addicted to a chemical substance or alcohol imbalance will occur.

We live with our memories everyday. We all live with the consequences of our actions. There are some actions that make us feel guilty and others, which cause us to feel resentment toward others. We need to be kind to our self and others. We do this by authentically forgiving our self and others, knowing that our actions and those of others were all that was available given the understanding of the moment. We can't change our past but we can change our view of it and understand it no longer needs to be relevant in our life. Live in the moment. Forgiveness!

Wipe the slate clean (the memory bank) through recognition and awareness. Start new from today with new attitudes and new ways of responding to one another. When we feel good about our actions, we can be happy and have feelings of wellbeing.

Things are not always, what they appear to be:
We always think everyone else is doing so well, forget it! It is never the case. Others may in fact be as apprehensive, insecure, yet may appear so self-assured and well off. Everyone has insecurities. We all have problems to one degree or another. We envision things with such fantasy. get over it! No one comes through life unscathed. It is only in our thinking, because we cannot see their life from their perspective. So believe it, no one has the perfect life.

Dealing with Anxiety
Whatever you are feeling do not fight it, flow with it, it is okay, it is not so terrible what you are feeling at the moment.

133

It is the fear of what is happening that makes it so terrifying. It is not actually the experience of anxiety, but rather the fear of it. Now, once we understand this aspect of the attack we can begin to bring it down to its proper perspective and see what happens to us at-the-moment, realistically rather than feeling so overwhelmed.

So, we begin by understanding the anxiety for what it is, and we come to understand that the anxiety itself is okay and often very normal, but it is the fear that we experience that is abnormal. The fear comes from believing we are the only person in the world to ever have felt or thought this way.

What we have to know is that others too have had the same thoughts, desires, feelings, and they are not so unusual. But, when our emotions are balanced, and we happen to have a strange thought or sensation, we shrug it off and do not become intimidated by it. And it is usually gone as quickly as it came. This is very normal, however, the fear that an agoraphobic feeds into it is not normal. And it is this fear that keeps us spinning on the cycle of fear until it becomes bigger than we can handle. We feel as though it is consuming our very being.

Letting Go Recovering from Agoraphobia
You can recover from agoraphobia. You may have indeed been a victim of circumstances and situations, but you must let go of the past and forgive it. You must decide if you will be a victim or a victor. And you do have a choice.

You have a choice to start living in the now for today and enjoy your life. You only have this moment in time, yesterday is past and gone and tomorrow is a new day. Make the best of it and learn how to live every day to the fullest and for yourself. If you are not good to you, you will not be good to others or your children. Sincerity is important, with God all things are possible but, with God sincerity is the basis to all things!

This is life's process and lessons. How will one know true appreciation until we have experienced the other side of joy and happiness? Until we know sorrow and pain. What would we have to compare it to? Would we know any different? Do we take our blessings for granted? Would we get the lesson otherwise?

Coming to terms

Stop analyzing everything. Come to terms with life and let it be through prayer.

It is necessary only to understand our past so that we may forgive it. Hand it over and be done with it. Put the past to rest and get on with your life. The old passes away and the new is the person we are today.

Face the present reality and the past

Face our history and allow our self to feel the pain, its not easy. For most people dealing with agoraphobia there is generally some type of addiction present in families, either with others or our self. Although it may not be evident, it is in the family of origin somewhere, perhaps in generations past but, it is there. At first, we deny this. Reach out to available resources and get into an environment that is supportive of our particular circumstances.

Using the tools that are available to us

Counseling, support groups, and prayer: Counseling is a tool, which helps you to gain perspective in your thinking. In counseling, we begin to understand what it is that we must face. The process helps us to let go of the old perspective, and forgive the situations that have wounded our minds and scarred our souls. It is not a cure but, a beginning.

Getting involved

When it is possible to do so, start to get out of your self by become involved with others. Join a church or spiritual group or join a 12 step group and start to use phone therapy as a means of reaching out to others.

Environment

If it is not conducive to well being and recovery, change it, whatever it takes. Changing attitudes a temporary reprieve. Talk, talk and talk to someone that you trust and can work with. Try to get out and do something that will build your self esteem.

Desensitize

Becoming exposed to and let surface the very things that cause fear. Work with a therapist in what I call pro-active therapy, it is almost like aversion therapy you are exposed to the source of your fear. This is very important. I cannot stress this enough, work with someone in these areas. The fear is usually masking the real problem. It is never what you think it is, always, completely different than what is apparent. Talk, talk and talk, this is how we resolve conflicts in our life and work through our feelings and emotions. Talk, talk, talk, the more we discuss them in a healthy way...the less power our feelings have.

The most important things that I have learned through re-covery

Let go of what you hide and that will be the beginning of a new and healthy you.

If we would take the time to research and review Gods way rather than hearsay, or distorted opinions, we would find a whole new world of blessings and knowledge. Do not stifle personal growth through doctrines or opinions.

We are missing life's pleasure in the trivial pursuit of being perfect. Everything is perfect, not in a human way, but in a God way. Humanity hasn't any ability to be perfect.

When we are controlling others lives, we are depriving them the challenge of meeting their own responsibilities

It is important to express with dignity our feelings, with as much respect for others and ourselves as possible.

I came into this world alone...I am responsible for only me.

The ESP of life emotional, spiritual and physical wellbeing and balance. It is not necessary to analyze everything, but, it is necessary to come to terms with it and let it be put the past to rest through prayer and meditation.

I do not believe that we can get well without realizing the need for a higher power (God) in our life and also to be able to forgive. This is imperative! It will be a challenge and is the key to our healing.

It is necessary only to understand our past, so that we may then forgive it. With God all things are possible but, with God sincerity of the heart is the basis to all things!

We have been affected as small children from generation-to-generation through distorted attitudes. It is the reason for our bitterness, anger, and resentment that we often feel as adults and for the loneliness that cannot be explained.

In coming to understand God in my life and his true nature, I am beginning to see that he is the essence of true acceptance.

We will be healthier and balanced human beings when we accept others and ourselves without all the prerequisites of what should" be and simply just live and let live and let it be.

We need flexible balance and structure to obtain a healthy existence, not rigid code and ethics, rules, and regulations. If your heart is not in it, it will mean nothing. When we are truly open to Gods spirit knowledge, understanding, and wisdom begins to fill our life and we come to know our purpose.

Afterword

I have come to know and understand things that in the years before my depression I had yet to see. And before I battled overwhelming anxiety attacks and "agoraphobia" I was totally unaware of, but as it happened, I had no choice but to search for a way to get well. In my desperation, I would have done anything to change what was happening....I was isolated and housebound for years.

As a result, I sought every available source of information and every avenue of cure......I researched, reviewed and debated information that was available and found a wealth of knowledge that is indisputable. Many of us have been misinformed concerning religion, spirituality, sexuality and addictions.

Consequently bitterness can become a way of life that destroys our very being and our spirits are in rebellion as to what is truth. It is my hope that in sharing life's "simple" truths, as I have come to know them.... that it is a blessing to others as well.

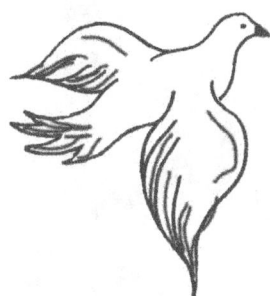

www.ingramcontent.com/pod-product-compliance
Lightning Source LLC
Chambersburg PA
CBHW072255270326
41930CB00010B/2385